Caroline Porter Thomas

PRAISE FOR

HOW TO SUCCEED IN NURSING SCHOOL

"Insightful and practical guide that will assist nursing students in successfully navigating their way through the wonderful and challenging world of nursing school."

Colleen Delaney PhD, RN, AHN-BC, Professor, University of Connecticut

"Caroline Porter's debut book 'How to Succeed in Nursing School' is an invaluable resource that offers sage advice and wonderful insight into the harrowing academic journey that is nursing school. I would personally recommend this jewel of a book to anyone who is considering nursing as a career or who has already begun their journey to the wonderful world of nursing. Those individuals who are considering becoming a nurse may not at first understand the difficulty of nursing school and may not see the value in Ms. Porter's advice but as a previously successful nursing student who graduated with academic honors from her nursing program and as a current registered nurse, I would advise that these words of wisdom be taken to heart. I would like to wish each and every individual who picks up this book the best of luck on their journey to becoming a nurse."

Gela D. Spivey, RN, Sanford, NC

"I found the suggestions and comments both positive and practical. The writing is very persuasive, since it is the product of Caroline's personal experience. These thoughts would be valuable for students working in many disciplines. This is a manuscript which is both helpful and wise. I wish Caroline Porter every success as the future unfolds." Walter J. Stohrer, S.g., Chaplain, Marquette University College of Nursing

Caroline Porter Thomas

HOW TO SUCCEED IN NURSING SCHOOL
BEFORE, DURING, AFTER

Caroline Porter Thomas, BSN, RN

Caroline Porter Thomas

Disclaimer

None of the information contained in this book should be construed as a claim or representation that you will be successful in gaining acceptance into nursing school or passing your nursing classes. The advice offered in the book personally helped Caroline Porter Thomas.

Publishing information: EmpoweRN

For information about special discounts for bulk purposes, please contact Caroline directly at (919) 721-2661 or empower.rn@gmail.com.. She is also available to speak at your institution.

Manufactured in the United States of America

ISBN-13: 978-1467950251

Caroline Porter Thomas

EmpoweRN.com

Where we focus on how we can be better nurses!

Tune in regularly for inspiration

Caroline Porter Thomas

Acknowledgments

This book is dedicated to the men and women who chose nursing as their profession in order to serve others during their times of greatest need. It is also dedicated to my parents Bruce and Ginger Porter. Mom you have an inspiring "get it done" attitude and Dad, you always encouraged me to use my imagination and have goals. Without both of your help and encouragement, this book would not be possible. I love you two so much and thanks for believing in me.

Special thanks to the professors at my Alma Matter Fayetteville State University. Specifically, professors Mary Dickey and Laura Pressley. I am so thankful for the excellent training I received. Your willingness and effort to answer my many questions was sincerely appreciated.

I would also like to thank my colleagues at Central Carolina community hospital. In particular, Elizabeth Tysinger for offering me my first job as a nurse. Also, Teresa Haigler for always seeing my potential and knowing when to challenge me. In addition, Linda Buchanan for always taking a minute or two to assist me. Also, for the staff at Holy Cross Hospital. Specifically Leola Saucier, Mary Jane Oppalano, Taj Singh and Nancy Rodriguez. You have made my time at this great institution truly enjoyable.

And most importantly, to my soul mate and best friend Emmanuel. Since I first saw you at the airport, our life together has been magical. I am so grateful to have you by my side. I love you.

Caroline Porter Thomas

CONTENTS

Foreword by Dr. Emmanuel Thomas

Introduction

Part 1: Before

Part 2: During

Part 3: After

Foreword

I am very excited about the arrival of the first edition of this book in 2011. It is a year of particular significance as healthcare reform is taking hold of the United States and nowhere will this impact be more felt than on nurses. Nurses are the lifeblood of medicine and with a universal plan that will give healthcare to most in America, nurses will be more in demand than ever. If one looks to the future, imagine what these changes will bring. Current nurses will have more leverage to find the job of their dreams in this field. Nursing students can rest assured that the hard work they are putting in to do well in their classes will be rewarded by a sea of jobs waiting for them after graduation. Lastly, individuals considering joining the nursing profession can rest assured that there will be adequate financial support for nursing schools by their affiliated universities and through federal aid that will ease the burden of the cost of this rigorous educational endeavor.

Therefore, this book arrives at the perfect time. During a period when increased demand is arriving for nurses, an educational tool is provided here that will help current and future nurses in all aspects of their nursing education, training and career. Imagine how you will feel as you finish reading the last page of this book. If you are a current student who is struggling through nursing school, you will have tools, resources and strategies that you can implement right away to improve your performance. For individuals who are considering nursing school, you will have knowledge to select the right school for you and also to start school with proven strategies that will propel you to academic excellence. If you have recently graduated from school, you will have internalized information that will help you pick the best field of nursing and also how to design your lifestyle by picking the right work schedule for you.

Now, move forward years ahead when you have been a nurse for sometime. Imagine all the good you will accomplish by helping those sick people who desperately need your care. Also, feel the satisfaction you will have from knowing you have a job that really matters: a job that improves the lives of the sick individuals and their families through improvements in health. It is clear that the most important thing in life is health and it has been said that health equals wealth so what better way to give than to provide nursing care to those in need of it. In my humble opinion, we have been placed on this planet to give and there is no better way to give than to give the gift of health.

In the future, as healthcare is provided for many of the 300 million individuals in the country, the healthcare system will be utilized more than ever before. Physicians will be left managing more patients than in the past and it will be up to the nurses to actually deliver the care and monitor the patient to ensure that their health is improving. In addition, recent research has provided evidence of the existence of a mind-body connection that directly influences a patient health. Positive mental states and outlook can greatly aid in the speedy recovery of a sick individual and this is where a nurse can also provide significant assistance. By fostering a nurturing and supporting environment for the healing of the sick patient, recovery can be accelerated decreasing the cost of healthcare to the patient and for our country as a whole.

This book is ultimately provided to you so that you can get to the final destination envisioned for you right here. With the help of this book, you can achieve a career in nursing where you will greatly contribute to the care of the sick and to anyone in need of medical care. With the arrival of travel nursing, you can do this anywhere you want. You can also be satisfied knowing that you will have a secure job that will pay you well for the rest of your life. Lastly, you can also choose and work under the nursing schedule of your desire that will provide you the extra time needed to care for your family, friends and to make ALL of your dreams come true. In the end, the author wants you to be able to live the life you have always wanted, wherever you want, and this book can help you do it by helping you thrive as a nurse.

Emmanuel Thomas, MD, PHD

Bethesda, MD

How to Succeed in Nursing School

Introduction

In today's world, it takes a special kind of individual to take on the role of nurse and caregiver in the medical field. In fact, the concept of healthcare as a whole in America has become a controversial subject. Between managed care insurance plans, skyrocketing health costs, the current state of the economy and the futures of Social Security, Medicaid and Medicare being questionable, doctors, hospitals and health care institutions are burdened by the overwhelming need for reliable assistance and support that facilitates their abilities to provide even the most basic health care to the masses. As a result, the role of the nurse has changed in recent years and now more than ever, our devotion and dedication to the care of others is critical to the continued success of the practice of medicine throughout the world.

If you have opened this book and happen to be reading this introduction, chances are you are an individual who has chosen to pursue a career in nursing. It is a tremendous undertaking and I would like to both thank you for taking the time to read this book and applaud you for choosing to become a caregiver in the health care field. I made the same choice myself and I specifically wrote this book for you. It is my hope that it will serve as a practical guide in answering some of the most basic and common questions you may have now that you are considering a career in nursing.

Why We Choose Nursing as a Career

According to **Wikipedia**, nursing is defined as *"a healthcare profession focused on the care of individuals, families, and communities so they may attain, maintain, or recover optimal health and quality of life from birth to the end of life."* That is EXACTLY what we do and it is important for you to keep that in mind over these next few years of nursing school and throughout your career. Remember that you are one of the special and gifted individuals who have made the choice to pursue a career in a field that involves the care and welfare of others. Their lives will depend on your abilities, dedication and most importantly your compassion and empathy. With that in mind, it is my hope that through my personal experiences in this book, you will gain a better understanding of nursing as a whole, and have a clear road map to help you navigate your way through the education and licensing process and on to a rewarding and fulfilling career in nursing.

Caroline Porter Thomas

About This Book

The first section of this book is titled, "Before" and it examines the endless opportunities that a nursing license can provide and tips that would be helpful when applying to a program. The second part of the book, "During" provides you with information that will be helpful to you while you are in nursing school. Finally, the last section of the book, "After" guides you through graduation and passing the licensing board examination.

You will be given tips from 25 different nursing professors nationwide who will share with you their experiences and advice on what it takes to be a successful nursing student. These respected professors are currently part of the faculty at many different educational institutions that range from community colleges and state universities to prestigious Ivy League schools such as Yale and Johns Hopkins and the information they provide here is invaluable. I have also included testimonials from students, recent nursing school graduates and seasoned nurses to both inspire and motivate you throughout your rigorous and sometimes demanding schedule of nursing school education courses.

I hope that you will find this book to be both helpful and inspirational as you read along. I thank you again for choosing nursing as your career and I wish you luck in your pursuit. Enjoy the book.

Part 1

Before

Caroline Porter Thomas

Chapter 1

The Benefits of Being a Nurse

My initial inspiration to become a nurse came from my mother. I'm sure that does not surprise you. When I was a child my parents made the decision to home school my four brothers, my sister and me, and it was my mother who made the selfless choice to stay home and teach us. My parents also vowed to continue to home school us until the time came when *we* would choose to do otherwise. At age twelve I opted to leave the safety of my home schooling environment and enter the institutional education system. Over the next few years my younger brothers followed in my footsteps and joined me in the public school system. With no children at home to worry about my mother was able to reevaluate her own life and pursue *her* dreams and desires.

She chose to return to nursing part-time. This decision surprised me. Somewhere deep down inside I am sure I remembered my mother had been a nurse, but having her around and available to me constantly prevented me from thinking about what that really meant. Shortly after she made the decision to go back to work she landed a fantastic nursing position that just happened to offer a substantial salary. My family and I were surprised to see how easily someone who devoted twenty years of her life to a home and a family could make the transition back into the workforce.

Not only was my mother welcomed back to the nursing field with opened arms, but she was also bombarded with different opportunities. She had to sort through her options and decide which would work best for her and our family. Amazingly, she was able to choose the hours and days she desired to work. After carefully thinking it through and discussing her many options with my father, she finally accepted a position. How many other professions afford you the opportunity to re-enter the work force after not working in it for almost twenty years?

Helping Others

My nursing license has enabled me to have a completely different outlook on life and has instilled a sense of security in me I have never known before. Mother Teresa once said, "We can do no great things, only small things with great love." Being a nurse gives me the opportunity to spread love to people every day and every minute I am on the job. Your view on life changes when you help others in need, when *you* are responsible for putting a smile on a patient's frowning face, when *you* are there at someone's life-altering moment. With these experiences you begin to realize the tremendous impact your small contribution and actions can have on those whose lives you touch.

Job Security

Nursing will not only fulfill a spiritual need but it will also offer you a degree of security. Knowing that no matter what stage of life you are in, where you live, what hours you have available to you, the fact that as a nurse you can always have a job if you want it or need it is priceless. In today's world such job security is rare. Just having a college education in America, which we are all so vested in as a society, does not necessarily guarantee the same success that it did in previous years. Too often we see people with bachelor's degrees in no better position than those with high school diplomas. Sometimes even a master's degree doesn't assure you of work. Many industry employers want to hire people who have experience in their field. This eliminates new graduates from the candidate pool.

It is not only the educational system that has changed, it is our society as a whole. In our grandparents', or even our parents' day, the definition of "living a good, productive life" involved working for a good company, advancing in position, and, through diligence and hard work, being able to provide a good life for your family. Then, when you reached your *"golden years,"* you retired on a

company pension and Social Security. Today, with huge corporations going bankrupt, the instability of Social Security, corporate pension funds and the stock market, such promises are limited.

Although a nursing degree will not solve every problem related to job security and retirement, it is a degree that allows you to have more control over your life by presenting you with options. I have many friends who graduated with their degrees and are still unemployed months and even years later. I also have friends who were never able to find work in their fields and were therefore forced to accept jobs unrelated to their degrees. I wanted to be sure my hard work and expensive education would pay off. I also understood that the medical profession fills a need, whereas many other professions fulfill wants. Let me describe the many nursing roles that are available, and you will have a better understanding of what I am saying here.

A Variety of Opportunities and Choices

Possessing a license in nursing provides you with a plethora of choices. You can choose to work in obstetrics and be part of that special moment when women give birth, or you can even choose to work in the newborn nursery. You can work directly with young children in pediatrics if that's your preference, or on the general medical floor where adult patients are admitted. If you are passionate about geriatric care you could serve the elderly community in a nursing home. With so many choices you do not have to make a decision immediately.

Hospitals alone offer numerous options. For example, in the private hospital where I work, there are two medical-surgical floors, a pediatric section, pre-intra-and post surgical sections, an intensive care unit and the emergency department. You could learn how to insert PICC lines, assist during radiological procedures, or work in dialysis. The list of opportunities goes on and on.

Large hospitals have even more nursing positions, with many more units to fill, such as specialized intensive care units (ICUs). Each surgical ICU, cardiac ICU, neurological ICU, and neonatal ICU, has its own step-down unit. The difference between the ICU and the step-down unit is the nurse to patient ratio and the complexity of the patient's illness. The ICU is typically one-to-one (one nurse per patient), or one-to-two. In the step-down units, the ratio is usually one-to-three (one nurse per every three patients). Of course, you cannot forget many of the larger hospitals have trauma units as well. All of these units have potential employment opportunities for the registered or licensed nurse.

Another good thing to know is that if you work in a unit or floor in a hospital and then realize it does not meet your expectations you can always switch to a different area of the hospital. It is not unusual for nurses to switch units or hospitals every one to three years. In some cases this may be encouraged because it provides you with range of different experiences which makes your resume appealing and also shows your versatility.

If you have trouble finding your niche and do not want to commit to any one particular section of the hospital then the float pool may be for you. This position is typically reserved for nurses who have at least one year of experience. In the float pool you are familiarized with many different floors of the hospital and thus work wherever needed. An added bonus is that you are generally paid higher wages than the regular staff nurses, and you can personalize your schedule. One disadvantage is that if the floor census (number of patients) changes you are almost always the first to be sent home. Benefits frequently are not offered with this position.

Flexibility

Flexibility truly is one of the best benefits of obtaining a nursing license. Nurses generally work three twelve-hour shifts per week. That means you have more than half the week off! Very few jobs offer such flexibility. If, however, you prefer to work eight-hour shifts, that is also an option. Many hospitals even allow short four-hour shifts, which are especially accommodating to young mothers. Here are a few examples of hospital shifts typically available to working nurses:

7 a.m. to 7 p.m.

7 p.m. to 7 a.m.

1 p.m. to 1 a.m.

3 p.m.to 3 a.m.

Eight-hour shifts usually are 7 a.m. to 3 p.m., 3 p.m. to 11 p.m., or 11 p.m. to 7 a.m. But these schedules can be negotiable. Some positions have a typical Monday through Friday schedule of 8 a.m. to 4 p.m. Although it may take some time to find the right position for you, you have much more flexibility to create a schedule that fits your life.

Most hospitals are flexible, depending on the department where you work, and will offer you a fixed schedule. There are options such as working three days during the week and then getting a long weekend. If you have children and need to be home during the week, you can work only weekends. This gives you the luxury of being available for all your child's ballet, soccer, and band practices. Having time off and a flexible schedule allows you to spend more time with those who matter to you most.

Since hospitals operate 24 hours a day, seven days a week, 365 days a year, employers are constantly looking for individuals who are willing to work night shifts. From my experience there are many benefits to working this shift. I noticed I was more able to focus on the tasks at hand during the less hectic atmosphere of the night shift. During the day there is a lot of activity in the hospital. Most days you will juggle doctor's visits, various tests such as x-rays and EKG's, and visitors. This activity can make your job stressful because it distracts you from completing your basic duties. At night, although you are still faced with some of the same challenges, the constant traffic is much less, and you have more time to concentrate on patient care and reporting.

Monetary Benefits

Another benefit of being a nurse is the opportunity to work extra shifts. Additional hours can be very lucrative for you. Some hospitals do not offer incentives or overtime so this does not apply to all places of employment. However, there are some hospitals that just cannot seem to get enough of you! As an incentive they offer a higher hourly rate, additional bonuses, and overtime pay once you have exceeded 40 hours in one week. I've experienced all three of these benefits first-hand. On several occasions, I earned almost $300 above my usual salary for 12 hours of work. Within my first six months of employment as a registered nurse I was able to take three out-of-state vacation trips that were completely financed with my overtime pay!

Vacation time is a major perk of being a nurse. Imagine starting a new corporate job in an office and asking for vacation time after two months of employment. As a nurse, you are able to make up your time off with extra shifts. After being employed as a nurse for only two months I took my first week-long vacation, and it cost me absolutely no vacation time what-so-ever. Nursing really rocks!

Traditionally nursing has been a profession dominated by women. However, it is now common to see men entering the field so the demographic of the "stereotypical" nurse shifted significantly in recent years. Broader salaries and the overwhelming need for responsible caregivers may have something to do with this shift. In the past, those who pursued nursing as a career were viewed as true philanthropists who chose to help others rather than work in more traditional or lucrative fields with higher salaries. Today nursing has become the lucrative career as salaries for nurses increased dramatically over the past few decades. The U.S. Bureau of Labor Statistics reported the average annual wage for registered nurses in 2006 was $57,280. If you consider the benefits and the amount of time you will have off in comparison to a typical job, that's a nice chunk of change for the investment.

Where You Can Make a Difference as a Licensed Nurse

So far, we have only discussed employment opportunities at hospitals, but keep in mind that being a nurse means there are many other options available for employment.

- You can work for any public health department in preventive medicine and focus on keeping people well as opposed to helping them recover.

- You can work in a private doctor's office or you could work for hospice and help individuals pass in comfort and dignity.

- Nurses work in the psychiatric field or conduct physicals as underwriters with an insurance company.

- There are numerous opportunities in outpatient surgical centers and even within the public and private school systems as a school nurse.

- Home health care is another option if you are comfortable in a home setting.

- Pharmaceutical and medical supply companies are constantly on the lookout for consultants.

- If you like adventure, you could be a flight nurse.

- If you wanted to serve your country and get great nursing and leadership experience, you could join the military.

- There are even opportunities to work from home as a nurse. There are jobs for research nurses and nurse educators.

The above list is by no means complete but it gives you a basic understanding of many opportunities awaiting you once you have a nursing license.

The Need for Nurses

I realize it can be a scary proposition to spend two to four years in school only to find there are limited positions available to you in your field once you have graduated. The good news is that this scenario is highly unlikely for nurses as the need for medical care assistance increases yearly. The U.S. Bureau of Labor Statistics recently said the future outlook for overall job opportunities for registered nurses is expected to remain high, but may vary by geographic location. In fact, the employment rate for RNs is expected to increase faster than all other occupations through 2016 with registered nurses projected to generate 587,000 new jobs in the U.S. alone. Additionally, hundreds of thousands of opportunities will open up as result of the numbers of experienced nurses projected to retire and/or leave the occupation. So rest assured that once you complete your educational requirements a great job will be waiting for you!

Caroline Porter Thomas

Chapter 2

Where Do You Start?

I hear it said all the time, "I want to be a nurse." To the average layperson, there may be nothing wrong with this statement and they may think it will be an easy process. But honestly, the process of becoming a nurse is complicated. There are several different types of nurses ranging from LPN and RN to BSN. The education requirements for all *are* similar, yet different in ways I will explain as we proceed. The following section will give you basic guidelines of the different ways you can become a nurse. You can use this section to evaluate your current status and better determine which path is best for you.

Licensed Practical Nurse or LPN

Advantages

- Only requirement is a high school diploma to enter a program.

- The course takes about a year to accomplish so you could be in the workforce soon.

- Programs are held at vocational centers and technical schools and also many high schools have special programs for practical nursing education. (These students receive their high school diploma and are immediately able to sit for the PN boards.)

- Entrance requirements are less and test scores can be lower than scores needed for RN schools.

- Depending on the program, you may or may not have prerequisites (although I highly recommend taking science classes like anatomy and physiology first). Stepping stone programs to get your RN are easily found.

- Other programs advertised are LPN to RN, LPN to BSN, and now LPN to MSN.

Disadvantages of LPN

- If your program requires prerequisites it may take you one to two years to complete them.

- Your scope of practice as an LPN is limited as some of your nursing documentation will have to be cosigned by an RN.

- Additionally, some of your nursing procedures must be started by an RN. For example, at my hospital LPNs cannot begin blood transfusions or perform initial patient assessments.

- Less pay for almost the same amount of work that RNs are required to do.

- From what I have witnessed, there seem to be fewer job offers, and it is especially difficult to get hired in most specialty care areas.

- If you already have a bachelor's degree in another field you may be limiting yourself by entering the nursing profession at a lower level (see accelerated program to BSN).

- Many of your previous science courses may expire after 5 or 10 years and you may have to repeat them (applies to all levels of nursing).

Associate Degree Nurse or ADN

(This program is designed to prepare you to take the RN boards.)

Advantages

- This program usually focuses more on technical nursing skills than nursing theory, the focus of BSN programs.

- You usually get this degree at a community college.

- It takes two years or 4 to 5 semesters.

- You can sit for the RN boards in two years versus getting a four-year university education and taking the same state boards.

- You have more marketability than an LPN.

- You enter the nursing workforce at a higher salary than an LPN.

- You have more opportunities for career progression.

- There are many RN-BSN programs available, which means an associate degree nurse can enter a program and have his or her BSN in about a year.

- Your education in general will be less expensive because it is at a community college.

- Many employers offer tuition reimbursement.

- Normally the student to faculty ratio is smaller.

- In many hospitals you can go into administration with your ADN.

- In many hospitals you can become a charge nurse.

Disadvantages

- You may have up to one year of prerequisites that need to be completed depending on your high school education.

- There may even be prerequisites for the RN to BSN program.

- Some hospitals now require you to have a BSN.

- Many associate degree programs require a CNA license before you apply or begin the program.

Diploma RN

Advantages

- Takes 3 years.

- Administered in a hospital.

- A diploma program requires students to do more clinical work than degree seeking students. Thus the adjustment into a permanent nursing position is usually easier.

- Hiring advantages exist because you are familiar to the hospital.

Disadvantages

- Many of these programs do not offer college credits that will transfer to a university, so if you want to progress to a BSN you might have to repeat some courses.

- There are only about 70 of these programs in existence today according to the

U.S. Department of Labor.

Bachelor of Science in Nursing (BSN)

Advantages

- Many employers favor an applicant with a BSN degree.

- This will open many positions in inpatient and community settings and will help you on the road to becoming an advance practice nurse.

- The educational focus trends more toward leadership roles with extensive training that prepares you for administrative positions.

- For many high school students planning to get a four-year degree, nursing offers an excellent career opportunity.

- Specialization requiring graduate level studies is easier. When you decide which advanced degree you want you can go directly to it (some programs may still require prerequisites depending on your school's undergrad course load.)

Disadvantages

- More expensive.

- Takes longer.

- Your first two years of school are not nursing centered and high grades in this non-nursing coursework are essential in order to get accepted to a nursing program.

- You may complete these two years and might not gain acceptance into the

  nursing program, as many programs are extremely competitive.

- Quite often your pay is the same as the ADN.

Accelerated BSN

Advantages

- If you have a bachelor's degree in another field you can apply to the program and obtain a BSN in 12-18 months.

- This is the fastest way to get into the nursing field if you already have a bachelor's in another field.

Disadvantages

- A 3.0 GPA is usually required.

- Prerequisites may apply, especially if you do not have a science background.

- There are only approximately 200 programs in existence, so you may have difficulty finding a program near you.

Researching Schools

When you decide which option is best for your career plans you can research schools in your area that offer appropriate courses. Using a Google search online you can go to your state's board of nursing website. For example, search for "Alabama Board of Nursing" and you'll find a section on the website listing approved nursing programs. Once you find schools offering nursing courses in your area continue researching to determine which one will be best for you. Some data and statistics you should pay particular attention to are:

- The school's accreditation.

- The school's acceptance and pass rates.

- Acceptance requirements.

You may have to call the schools and speak to someone in the nursing department to get this information.

Accreditation will be either through the NLN (National League of Nursing) or the CCNE (Commission on Collegiate Nursing Education). Accreditation is important especially if you want the option to pursue your master's degree later (advanced degrees will be discussed in the last chapter). There are nursing programs that are approved by the board of nursing which may not be accredited. If you are looking only to work as a nurse, an unaccredited school may be your best option. Acceptance into a nursing program at any school can be challenging. Sometimes schools that are not accredited have less demanding admission requirements than those that are accredited.

What You Will Need

It's important for you to get statistics on a school's acceptance rate and grade point averages. For example, find out how many of the school's graduates actually started the program at that institution from the beginning. If a school starts out with 50 students in their program, but only graduates 9, that should be a consideration in choosing the school. Are those the kinds of statistics you want to be part of? Be aware that some of these programs proudly say their students have a 100% pass rate of the NCLEX boards without taking into account some of these variables. I believe that it is better to go to a school with a lower pass rate than to risk failure midway through the program offered at other schools boasting perfect pass rates. Once you graduate you may take the board examination several times if you need to.

Knowing the school's acceptance requirements is important because, along with prerequisites, many schools have additional requirements to gain acceptance into their programs. One of the most common is the Nursing Entrance Exam (NET). The NET applies to all nursing levels. You will need to study for this because the questions center around basic math, reading, and comprehension skills. Score requirements for admission differ from school to school and are only valid and applicable for a certain amount of time depending on the school. Your particular score may only be applicable for six months to a year. So if you have a year or more of prerequisites you do not want to take the test too early.

It is imperative that your score be relatively high because some schools will make you wait up to one a year before allowing you to re-test and may limit the number of times you can repeat it. Due to the variety of different tests available "good" scores are dependent upon which test you take. Be sure to find out what score is acceptable depending. That's why it's important for you to study because you may not get another chance to improve your score. You can find study books and prep tools online, or at your local book store. Be sure to ask the school's nursing department which particular book they recommend for test preparation.

The minimum GPA requirement is another thing to consider as you complete your prerequisites. The school may advertise that you must have a minimum cumulative GPA of 2.5, but because nursing school is competitive and many schools have waiting lists for only a few slots, you may want to strive for a much higher GPA.

Of the required prerequisite courses, make sure your science and math grades are very good. Nursing is a science, after all, and strong grades in these subjects are a basic foundation and can determine how well you will do in upper division nursing. Only with an understanding of normal anatomy and physiology will you be able to comprehend complicated disease processes and treatments.

Many schools require a Certified Nursing Assistant (CNA) license before you apply. This certification is offered at many community colleges and generally takes about two to three months to complete. Some schools consider whether you worked as a CNA in order to determine if they will accept you or not, so it is good to have about six months of experience doing this. It is possible for you to get this experience while you are completing your prerequisites by working part time if your schedule permits and your prerequisites aren't too demanding.

All of this information may seem overwhelming as you consider which program is right for you and determine where to attend school. But remembering the reasons you decided to pursue nursing will keep the challenges in perspective. Here is the personal journey story of Bailey Evans, who shares her reasons for becoming a nurse. Bailey discusses the challenges she faced in school and offers hope and encouragement to nurses at the beginning of their careers.

Bailey's Story

"When I was seven, I did a cartwheel down the living room stairs and put my little brother in a body cast. Legs, leotard, and pigtails flailing, I smacked right into him and fractured his femur. I pulled him around the block in the old red wagon every day during his recovery. One time I even helped him get a Cheeto out of his cast.

"I have not always wanted to be a nurse and breaking my brother's leg did not result in a revelation. I was just a kid, and I was actually really freaked out by anything medical. My fear of getting the board game Operation as a gift even caused me to call off my birthday party. I could just see myself ripping away the wrapping paper only to find that man with the clown nose staring up at me, begging me to remove his 'spare ribs.' No, thank you.

"When I was a sophomore in college, I made the decision to go to nursing school. I guess I wanted to challenge myself to see if I could actually really do something in life that seemed to scare the living daylights out of me. Previously on the track toward social work, I knew I had a love for people's stories and wanted to do more to help. Being the first in my family to enter the medical profession,

How to Succeed in Nursing School

I had no idea what I was getting myself into. In fact, I sort of just went with it, knowing that no matter where I ended up in life that nursing school would teach me a lot about myself. The more I went along, learning about nursing and spending time with patients, the more I fell in love with this incredible profession.

"People always want to know why I chose nursing school over medical school. A doctor drops by, solves the symptoms puzzle and heads out the door. It is the nurse's job to stick around to help the patient cope. Good nurses take time to treat the illness and the individual: fielding concerns, providing comfort, training patients in self-care. I always laugh when my friends ask me if medical television shows depict the way life really is in a hospital. You mean, when they show a handsome stud doctor drawing a.m. labs and then pan out to a nurse rolling a patient's wheelchair down the hall in the background? Any nurse will tell you that image is hilariously false, except maybe the part about the doctor being a stud. But really, I love to explain to people what nurses do and how important nurses are. One of the first things I tell people is that nurses must have the ability to communicate with everyone, period. They even kind of have to be telepathic sometimes.

"As a nursing student, the ability to communicate and integrate myself into the healthcare team has not come easy for me. The thought of reporting my findings to doctors still makes my stomach turn, but I am thankful for the great deal of practice I have received in clinical. I learned very quickly that you cannot be timid in nursing school. My instructors had this shy wallflower throwing back the sheets and examining every inch of a patient's skin for evidence of breakdown on day one. At the time, I thought they were putting me through some kind of cruel nursing student initiation, but now I am able to walk into a patient's room and discuss the plan of care for the day without batting an eyelash, I thank them for forcing me to take giant leaps out of my comfort zone every day.

"Nursing school has given me courage in every aspect of my life. I cannot tell you how many times I have been faced with awkward social situations, or the need to make a tough phone call, or the chance to do something really difficult or scary, and I've told myself, 'Man, if I made it through clinical this week, I can make it through anything.'

"As an academic peer tutor for my nursing school, I have had the opportunity to work with and mentor many new nursing students. Their fears are the same as mine, and are shared by many. The best help I ever received is the knowledge we are not alone out there. Even if it seems like we are sometimes – when everything in clinical is going wrong, when our patient does not like us, when our preceptor nurse is cranky, when we keep drawing a blank with important things we need to know – even then we are not alone. Take a quick look down the hall of any school or hospital. Every nurse and every nursing student you see has gone through or will go through what you are experiencing now. It is not unusual, and you can take comfort in the fact there will always be someone there to empathize with you and offer you support.

"When I was 20, when I was accepted into the professional nursing program, I would sit in the library and 'gross out' my engineering and Spanish literature friends by rattling off course objectives that included the words like 'catheter' and 'nasogastric.' Something about the idea of dealing with things that made other people squeamish always intrigued me. Yes, I knew I wanted to be one of the people who did all of the 'dirty work,' but it was more than that. I knew I wanted to take care of people and their families at some of the most critical times in their lives.

"Back when I was seven, while my brother was in the hospital with his Ninja Turtles cast up to his belly button, I came down with strep throat. I was offered the option of taking a shot and being able to go in and watch cartoons with him, or taking a course of antibiotic pills and waving at him through the thick glass. For the first time in all of my seven years, I wanted a shot. You know what it feels like when you just know something is right for you? That's how I felt about that shot, and that's what nursing has become for me. It has been something I have grown into, and will continue to grow into as I progress and my career develops.

"I am 23 now and about to graduate with a bachelor of science in nursing. I'm excited, terrified, and proud of myself all at the same time. I have been through some of the most difficult, stressful times of my life, but every last tear and every rough day was completely worth it. Believe me, no one was more surprised about my decision to become a nurse than me, the shy kid who used to be afraid of hospitals. So you see, anything is possible."

Bailey Evans, BSN, RN
The University of Texas at Austin

Chapter 3

What You Need to Know Before You Start

By necessity there is a lot of material in nursing school. It is the job of the instructor to sort through it for the essentials (and after that there is still a lot).

Mary Brann, MSN, RN

Touro University

For those students who have gone straight to college from high school the transition from your prerequisites to nursing content will be easier. You are already in the swing of things, you have developed good study techniques, and have figured out your preferred learning style. Many of you live in dormitories or in your parent's house. Some of you however are older, returning to school after many years of being away. Many of you have bills to pay, mouths to feed, and houses to clean and tend to.

For the students with multiple responsibilities I would like to stress the importance of planning ahead. Even though you may have already completed your anatomy and physiology, chemistry, and statistics classes, I must point out that nursing school is entirely different. When I compared notes with friends in other majors there was absolutely no comparison in the workload. In my opinion, nursing school takes much more time and dedication than many other degrees.

To study for a nursing class means going above and beyond, further than you have gone for a class before. This is why if you have children, husbands, wives, or other responsibilities, I would highly encourage you to put some major time into planning before you take the plunge. I have known people in my nursing school with degrees in other disciplines who "flunked out" of the nursing program. There are three major areas of your life that you want to examine. They are:

- Your current financial situation
- The time commitment
- The emotional investment

Caroline Porter Thomas

Can You Afford it Financially and Emotionally?

Going to college is a huge financial burden for the student. I have no statistics to offer you as to the average debt of most students but I do know this. I personally graduated with about $27,000 worth of debt, and that was a low amount of money compared to my peers and classmates. Of course, this number is subjective depending upon where you attend, how many years it takes to graduate, and which degree you pursue. Regardless, education is not cheap.

It is important to determine cost of living while you are in nursing school. I encourage you to make a plan for yourself before you even start. The plan could be to live with your parents as they help support you, or you could work for a full year before you even start to save money. My plan involved moving back in with my parents so I would not have too many bills. To subsidize, I took out as many student loans as I could, but still had very little extra money to play around with. Planning for your financial future could mean the difference between being able to focus on your studies easily and being completely stressed out about money and the possibility of it running out before you finish school.

You may have no other choice but to work while you are a student nurse. Many nursing students work as CNAs (certified nursing assistants) in hospitals or nursing homes while in school. It is good to have at least six months experience before you even start nursing school. While this prepares you for full-time work in a healthcare environment, I personally feel this job can be stressful physically and emotionally. The workload in general is very heavy and may be too much for you to take on while attending nursing school. As a nurse I have often seen private sitters reading or studying for hours while their patients sleep. Consider or seek other options that have the potential to be less stressful and allow you the time to read or study.

Before you even start nursing school it would be in your best interests to look for a less demanding job. Something like working at a dry cleaner or as a salesperson in retail for example. If you wanted to stay in the healthcare setting, consider telemetry monitor technician or phlebotomist. Jobs like these two would not give you study time, but you would be in the healthcare surrounding and it is not as physically or emotionally demanding as CNA work. Each of these will take a few months to get certified. In the end only you know what is best for you and what your limitations are.

With all of this in mind, if you have not started nursing school yet and you happen to be a person who already has responsibilities, I encourage you to think long and hard about the endeavor you are about to embark upon. Please be honest with yourself. Look at your life and where you are, and take action to make your experience better. If you are already in nursing school it may be difficult for you to take a step back and assess how much stress you are currently dealing with. But it is helpful to decide if stress is affecting your performance in nursing school. If you suspect this is the case, look for ways to make your life easier and less stressful as you go along. As I mentioned, moving in with your family as I did could alleviate financial stress. You could also consider taking out more loans or find other students in your situation and work together.

Too often we assume nursing school is going to be a struggle in many ways so we "bite the bullet" and prepare for the worst. We have all heard stories of how people have overcome extraordinary obstacles in order to complete their education. I have no doubt that anyone facing major obstacles who still manages to get their degree is an amazing person. The problem is that many people who are struggling in school find themselves unable to persevere and graduate. They simply give up because of the stress level. Plan ahead so you can be a successful nursing student!

Taking a few steps back in your life will be less tragic than you think. I will use myself as an example. I started my own retail business when I was 19 years old. I made enough money to live comfortably on my own, have a nice car, and travel to nine different countries throughout the world. I did this for three years until finances became tight, and I became physically ill from working so hard during the last year. This forced me to make some serious decisions as to how I would handle my future and the next chapters of my life. It was at that point that I decided to go back to school because I realized it would open many doors for me and help me to secure my future.

Change Creates Opportunities

When I started school, I began working at a restaurant making $30-$70 a day. I had been fortunate enough to secure a significant amount of money in student loans, but it still really wasn't enough money for rent, food, and my other bills.

I found myself picking up extra shifts at work so I could survive. As a result, my grades suffered my first semester back at school. I realized a "C" average was not good enough to get accepted to nursing school, and I needed to make some changes – and fast – because what I was doing was clearly not working. I asked my parents if I could move in with them. It wasn't an easy transition. Essentially I gave up my freedom, my job, my leisure time with friends, and more. In retrospect, now that I have finished nursing school, I undoubtedly made the right decision.

You have to ask yourself what changes you could make in your life that would better prepare you for nursing school. I have spoken in great length with many fellow students in my prerequisite anatomy and physiology (A&P) classes about this. They would always approach me because they wanted to know how I was getting A's while they were averaging C's and D's. When I explained it had nothing to do with smarts and everything to do with less stress and making my life less complicated, they would tell me it was a frustrating challenge for them to do the same. When I asked why, their responses were:

" I don't get along with my parents."

"My family member wants to know everything I'm doing."

"They can't accept the fact that I like to stay out late sometimes.

And so on and so forth.

Sadly, the majority of those students did not even make it through the A&P class.

If you find yourself relating to the unsuccessful students mentioned above I would like you to look at the facts. Nursing school requires a two- to four-year commitment and upon graduation numerous hospitals will be offering you jobs. Soon after passing your boards you will be making enough money to provide for yourself and those you are responsible for. Isn't the sacrifice of your freedom worth the outcome? The answer is yes, because by making the commitment and sacrifice you will gain much more freedom in the future.

I also speak with many people who really want to go to nursing school but do not want to take out student loans. Student loans are the best type of loan offered to people. They are low interest and payments are deferred until after graduation. Even if your credit is destroyed you can be approved for a low-interest student loan quickly and easily. What credit card company would give you $10,000 a year to complete your education in spite of your very low credit rating score? The reason that institutions offering student loans are flexible is because they know that once you graduate you will be able to pay them back easily. So why not apply and give yourself more money for food, gas, or rent?

Currently, my $27,000 in student loans require a monthly payment of about $230. Would you believe my employer actually pays for my student loan as an incentive for working for them? I realize not every job may offer this convenience, but many employers do. It is something to keep in mind.

Time Factors and Emotional Components

I won't lie to you. Nursing school is rigorous; it's demanding and time consuming. Nursing school requires many hours of clinical time; the number of hours varies depending on where you attend school. Most, if not all, of your classes will usually run late because there is so much information that has to be presented. With all you will have to learn, procrastination is not the study method of choice for nursing students (Believe me, I tried). You will need at least two to four hours of study time every day in addition to your clinical and class time.

And don't forget to consider the emotional component of attending nursing school. When I started nursing school I promised myself I would strive for and maintain a 4.0 grade point average. I achieved that for the majority of my prerequisites. The fact is, it is almost impossible to have a 4.0 grade point average in nursing school, and if you have ever seen a nursing school textbook you will understand why. Even my friends attending medical school frequently commented about how my books were impressive due to their size and massive amount of content. Nursing text books are overloaded with information to ensure students understand as much as possible. It is not uncommon for a review test to cover over six chapters of text. It's quite a bit to manage if you happen to have three to four classes at a time. Needless to say, the content reading requirements of nursing school can be overwhelming. That quantity of reading, combined with long clinical hours, make it difficult to always stay positive. No matter how strong you think you are, the stress could eventually put you on an emotional roller coaster.

Think Positively

Occasionally, things you perceive as negative experiences will happen to you. You may get a low grade on an exam, fail to perform a procedure properly or struggle with a complicated medical concept. Try to look at your low test score as a gift that reveals truths to you about areas where you need improvement. Do not give up because if you truly are persistent, you will succeed. Two things that helped me through those difficult times were positive books filled with quotes and videos that inspired me to persevere. I listened to people like Tony Robbins, Marci Shimoff, Deepak Chopra, and Joel Osteen, and they made a positive impact on my overall outlook. You have to admit that other people's wisdom can move you in some way. You can use these tools anytime you need an emotionally positive boost.

For additional reinforcement and motivation, I would like to present to you Baochau Elizabeth Nguyen's inspiring story. Like many of us, her decision to become a nurse was a passionate one filled with moments of trial and error.

Elizabeth's Story

"Volunteer. Student. Pre-medicine. Lost. Confused. Patient. Realization. Pre-nursing. Applications. Stress. Acceptance letter. Nursing. Confidence. Compassion. As strange as it may seem, those words in the first two lines have summed up my adventurous four years as a college student. I entered college feeling so sure I was going to medical school, but I found out that sometimes having a plan does not mean that it is set in stone. The walk of life will take you upon many hills and curves and occasionally, you travel down that road that makes your life just a little more tranquil.

"At the age of six, I had the ability to fix a broken heart, cure a charley horse, and could remove butterflies from the stomach. At the age of six, the popular Milton Bradley game Operation had ignited my interest for healthcare, but I had no idea where it would take me in life. Growing up, I had always watched medical shows such as E.R. and Doogie Howser M.D., but I could never understand the medical terminology that was spoken. Terms such as STAT and NPO were just random words that were spoken when I played doctor. When I finally turned fifteen, I decided to volunteer at a Houston-based hospital, Memorial Hermann Memorial City, and my interest for healthcare grew exponentially. As a volunteer, I was fortunate enough to work in different units around the hospital and meet people of all different ethnicities and backgrounds. When I went off to college, working in healthcare became more of a reality. With increased exposure to other hospitals as a college volunteer, I was beginning to have more patient-to-patient interaction. As I was exploring the different options in healthcare, I made the decision to pursue nursing when I thought about all the different people I had ever encountered.

"The turning point to pursue nursing came when I was volunteering one day. On the floor I was working, I spoke with an elderly woman about my career interests. We had a nice talk and in the end she stated, 'A smile goes a long way. Keep your smile and it will take you a long way, whatever you decide to do in life.' I realized then that I found more joy in watching a patient's health improve as time went on. I realized I wanted to be a nurse. Nurses are the individuals who care for patients from the day they walk through the doors of the hospital to the day they walk out those doors. This elderly woman helped me tremendously with my career choice. I was grateful for her assistance, but I wish I had the opportunity to thank her.

"It was approximately 1 ½ years ago that I decided to pursue a career as a nurse and to pursue my nursing education at the University of Texas at Austin. 'The man who has confidence in himself gains the confidence of others.' This Hasidic saying is a phrase I learned to live my nursing school life by. After completing my first semester and working at various clinical settings, I have seen the impact nurses have on patients. The heart of a nurse speaks above all else. But nursing school was not easy. I was taking 16 hours my first semester and was running on little sleep. Looking back at it now, I can see how much I have grown as a student nurse and how much I have accomplished. Despite getting little sleep, an encounter with a patient during my first semester reaffirmed that I was going down the correct career path. In all settings, patients want to be able to look up to their healthcare providers and know they are in good hands.

"In the academic setting, I had the opportunity to have a clinical at a rehabilitation hospital in Austin. Many of these patients had experienced total knee or hip replacements and many could not perform essential activities of daily living such as bathing, eating, dressing, or grooming. I remembered this one female patient who many nurses described as a 'trouble maker.' Although this is not a therapeutic form of communication given from nurses, I did not want their biases to affect how I would execute good nursing care. The patient had a history of alcohol and drug abuse and was recovering from not only a total knee replacement, but from withdrawal as well. She initially looked tired and upset. I introduced myself and continued to carry on with my nursing care plan of the day. I performed a total bed bath and made sure I paid attention to her hair and feet. After her bath, she looked up at me and stated, 'You have restored my dignity through the many tough days of healing ahead.' The confidence I had in myself as a student nurse inspired this patient to bestow her confidence in me, so I was able to assist with her care and recovery.

"My desire to become a nurse has also pushed me to set very specific goals for myself. My first aspiration is to graduate from the University of Texas at Austin with a bachelor's degree in nursing. My love for children initially fueled me to pursue pediatrics as my specialty when I graduated. After my first semester of nursing school and working as a nurse's aide this past summer, I discovered that I want to be an ICU nurse. Although these patients are extremely sick, I will be able to devote more time and true nursing care to them. Working on the ICU floor has been a challenge, but these patients truly put one's nursing skills and abilities to the test. After working on the floor, my second aspiration would be to continue my education and obtain my master's degree to become a nurse practitioner.

"As a student at the University of Texas, I have found a very rewarding activity that contributes to the nursing community. I recently started working at the School of Nursing Learning Center as a tutor. I am able to assist students with various pre-nursing and nursing courses that I have successfully completed. The task of helping other students learn material for their courses is not easy, but it has been a rewarding experience when they give me positive feedback about being successful in their classes as well.

"Recently, Hurricane Ike caused immense damage in the Texas gulf coast area. My family, along with millions of others in Houston, was affected by this hurricane. My parents had no electricity or water for two weeks. The School of Nursing provided students the chance to volunteer all over Austin to provide nursing care to evacuees. Being able to help out the community with the education I have obtained in nursing school so far has been the most rewarding experience possible. Although many are still recovering from this incident, I am fortunate that I was able to help.

"I write this to future nursing students, pre-nursing students, and to nurses around the nation to hopefully inspire others. Although nursing school is not easy, it is a worthwhile journey that will truly enrich your life. I am graduating in December and I can remember the day I was a pre-nursing student and started my first semester of nursing school. Most importantly, I learned to believe in myself and my ability to become a nurse and care for those who need my help.

"Confidence in one's abilities makes any venture possible. I still have a lot to learn in nursing school because it is far from over, but one semester always has the ability to make me feel like a new person in terms of what I can do as a student nurse. I found something I really enjoy doing with my life; the hurricane showed me how I can put my skills toward the greater good of the community. Each person has an ideal, a hope, a dream that represents who they are and what they believe in. I can only hope the confidence I portray will display as compassion, understanding, and encouragement to my patients.

"Even though I am close to ending one chapter in my life and starting a new one, I keep my morals and values near and continue to have confidence in myself and my abilities. I have learned that life truly is what you make it to be and even though I have a plan for myself, I have seen that sometimes you just have to follow wherever life may take you. From medical surgical to psychiatric to OB-GYN and pediatric clinical and courses, my last semester in the fall will truly be an accumulation of what I have learned these past four years. The synthesis of knowledge will only continue when I am out in the real world practicing as a nurse. As the Indian philosopher Patanjali said, 'When you are inspired by some great purpose, some extraordinary project, all of your thoughts break their bonds, your mind transcends limitations, your consciousness expands in every direction, and you find yourself in a new, great, and wonderful world. Dormant forces, faculties and talents become alive and you discover yourself to be a greater person than you ever dreamed yourself to be.''

Baochau Elizabeth Nguyan, BSN, RN
The University of Texas at Austin

Caroline Porter Thomas

Chapter 4

The Transition to Nursing Courses

The variability keeps me interested, whether it's a change in clinical area and skills to challenge me or other areas to grow in, like management or teaching. Nursing is never dull or boring.

Lynn M. Garrett, RN

Nurse for more than 20 years

Specialty: CCU and PACU

If you're like me, chances are that memorization skills probably got you through your prerequisite classes. Regardless of the fact, your nursing classes will require you to memorize information, you must also take the next step and be able to apply that knowledge. To give you an appropriate analogy, I want you to take a moment and journey back to high school algebra class where you were taught to memorize formulas and then plug in the numbers accordingly. You used the formula, arranged the numbers and then chose the correct answer. Nursing questions are presented in application format before you begin, and understanding that way of thinking will put you ahead of the game.

You may remember applying formulas to pass the tests, but do you remember every single formula you learned? I'm going to assume your answer is no, although there may be a few mathematicians who do. For most of us, even remembering two or three formulas can be a challenge. This is one of the reasons nursing school is difficult. A board of nurses must verify we are safe caregivers, and in order to do this efficiently and effectively, they test using extremely difficult, "application style" questions. This ensures students have retained what was learned in class. Remember, as a nurse you hold people's lives in your hands, and even simple mistakes can mean the difference between life and death for your patients.

The Importance of A & P

Now that you have an understanding of why you cannot simply memorize information, the next step is to understand why your anatomy and physiology is crucial in nursing school. The first section in each subject category in nursing text is a brief review of relevant A&P; however, A&P is an entire class on its own. If you have a clear understanding of the content portion of the A&P, you will be able to move on to the main topics of that section, which is the disease portion of the book or pathology.

It may be difficult to get familiar with every section of A&P. Assess the areas you need to review and always start by reading about it. You may need a little extra assistance, and I recommend going to your nursing instructor and asking them to describe the function to you. When a nurse works in a specific field for years, he or she learns a lot about pathology and the applicable A&P. As a nurse, you will constantly educate your patients and you must be able to break down medical terms and language into layman's terminology. This is yet another reason why nursing school classes are much more difficult than the prerequisite classes because we need to be in a position to educate the general public. This can be very challenging and takes quite a bit of patience and requires a true desire to help patients grasp the information.

The next thing I want you to understand is that your instructors cannot possibly teach you everything you need to know in order to pass nursing school and the NCLEX. Sometimes nursing students with 4.0 GPAs from good nursing schools do not pass the NCLEX. This is because massive amounts of nursing materials need to be presented, and there is not enough time to do it. An average nursing book can have thousands of pages and present hundreds of diseases, and teachers cannot create test questions only from the reading material. That would be too easy, and you would not have a complete understanding of all of the information required to be considered a competent nurse.

Consider the amount of time we have in each class. The average class is three credit hours a week. That equals approximately 150 minutes of class time dedicated to any particular subject. In three hours, your teacher is supposed to cover three to six chapters, when the average chapter can be up to 80 pages. You must understand that with so much information for you to absorb, this task is virtually impossible. Even the greatest of teachers cannot present all the material in all the chapters in a way that you would be able to understand them.

The bottom line: You must learn on your own. You must go above and beyond what you learn in class and read in your books. I heard this from day one in nursing school but had absolutely no idea of the truth of those words until further along in my career. I kept thinking that going above and beyond meant reading more and more books. I could not even finish the reading assignments with good understanding as it was, and I kept asking myself how they expected us to do this when they were giving us hundreds of pages to read at a time and just days to do it. There is a way, and it is a lot easier than you realize. I will share it with you later in Chapter 7.

The Power of Critical Thinking

If you were an instructor and were teaching someone that A+B=C, it would be an easy task. A+B will always equal C, no matter what happens. As you learn to be a nurse, facts need to be examined and calculated. There are so many different considerations in order for you to connect the right question with the right answer, and one simple word can make the difference between getting the answer right or wrong.

Essentially, it is our instructor's responsibility to teach us to think critically and not select the first answer that pops out at us when we are questioned. Read the question numerous times and then read each and every answer numerous times. Then think about the question and what it is specifically asking, considering the outcome of each possible answer. This is critical thinking at its best, and it takes a lot of brain power and focus to do it well. Your instructor only has the capacity to present methods and ways to implement those methods. You are the one who must follow through to do your job well.

An Easy Instructor May Not Have Your
Best Interests in Mind

In nursing school, you may come across an easy instructor. He or she will go over a few textbook sections every week or present similar questions and scenarios repetitively in test reviews. Be aware that there is nothing easy about nursing school, and that includes textbooks and test reviews. In the end, this nice teacher is not giving you what you need in order to be successful when you take the boards. As a rule, the easier the class is, the harder you must study on your own. Learn to appreciate your difficult or challenging nursing professors. The ones who have the hardest exams followed directly by huge reading assignments are truly looking out for your best interests. The professors who make you absolutely nuts and stressed out of your mind are the individuals you will owe thanks.

I have to tell you from experience the NCLEX is the hardest test I have ever taken. So essentially, your most difficult teacher is actually preparing you to pass your boards. Those instructors will help you learn how to think critically, without overlooking the obvious. They understand the road ahead of you is a tough one and that it will not serve you well if they make things easy. They also understand the nature of nursing, the way the real world functions and that nothing is black or white. The gray areas are numerous. Appreciate your difficult, impossible instructors. They are helping, not hindering. And most importantly, they are preparing you to do whatever it takes to pass the NCLEX.

A Note from Ginger

"If you are a nursing student now, you may be questioning your sanity and why you so willingly subjected yourself to this torture. I want to encourage you to keep moving forward, because in my opinion you will discover, as I have, that the price you are paying now is worth it!

"My story began many years ago at the young age of 17. I sat in the admission counselor's office at our local technical college, assuming I was to sign into the secretarial science program in order to continue advancing in this field, since I had taken business courses during my last year of high school and then worked a summer filing job with civil service. However, much to my surprise, she said, 'Your test scores are high. Would you like to enroll in our new associate degree nursing program?' So, after about 30 seconds of deep thought, I said, 'I will try it,' and, two years later I graduated with the first ADN class from Fayetteville Technical Institute in Fayetteville, NC, and took an RN position in the hospital.

"Next to marrying my husband, Bruce, this was the best life decision I have ever made. During our first years of marriage, I had several interesting RN jobs. He was a US Army officer on the fast track, which meant we moved often. I never had a problem getting a job. However, my focus was forced to change from RN to mommy six years later, once we started our family (which eventually produced six children). Somehow during this time, I was able to complete my BSN, working on it part-time for several years. At sometime during the children's formative home schooling years, I placed my license on 'inactive' status, not even thinking I would be able to return to work; actually wondering if I would ever get all these kids out of diapers! Yes, it is true you can actually leave the profession and come back when you are ready. The saga continued and somehow many, many years later I reentered the RN work force with little difficulty. How many other career fields would welcome you back with open arms after such an extended absence?

"I love nursing! As a nurse I am able daily to touch another in a meaningful way and to comfort the uncomfortable. Years of wonderful memories are speeding through my mind as I think of my nursing experiences. I encourage you to grab hold of this great opportunity to join a profession unlike any other. A profession where you, too, can make a difference! So if you are a student nurse, or a potential student nurse, be assured that all Caroline is telling you in this book is true; carry on, go for it, it is worth it!"

Ginger Porter, RN (My Amazing Mom)

Nurse for more than 20 years

Specialty: Emergency Department

Caroline Porter Thomas

Part 2

During

Caroline Porter Thomas

Chapter 5

Make the best use of your class time

My favorite thing about nursing is helping patients get better.

Chin Schramm, RN

Nurse for 10 year

Specialty: med-surg

I want to share with you tools that helped me make the most of my class time. If you use your class time wisely studying on your own will also be easier. When I was in nursing school I noticed that students who were successful, including me, were always prepared. I remember thinking, "If everyone knew how a little preparation could make such a dramatic difference, they would do it." While these steps are simple and easy to do, they're also easy not to do. However, when these simple steps are completed it will make your class time exponentially more valuable and possibly even more enjoyable.

To begin, look over the chapters by glancing at the content on the pages. Set aside about 30 minutes every four to five hours or three times a day and look at the bold words, pictures, and highlighted sentences. Nursing exams generally test on multiple chapters so it is important you start this process as soon as you can. Ideally, begin immediately after you have taken your last exam so you can get a head start on new material. This step helps you recognize the words and familiarizes you with the content. After several times of looking at a word read the definition. As you read the definition notice how you are able to focus on what the word means.

Doing this simple step can eliminate reading without understanding. We must see a word several times before our brain flags it as important. That is why after the third or fourth time you look over information you finally say to yourself, "Okay, I have heard and seen this several times and I must know more about it!" Once you have reached that point you will find yourself directing all of your attention to the word's definition. And that motivation is because you have seen it so many times. There is still a problem though, because in nursing school there are thousands upon thousands of words. By just reading you rely on vision to get you through and retain all of this knowledge. Although this is possible, and has probably worked in the past, this is not an ideal way to study for nursing classes.

After you look at the words and read the definitions a few times, go back and underline each word and definition. This helps you engage the body by adding movement. Then say the words and definitions out loud. Doing so engages the three senses of sight, touch, and sound. You are also using all three learning styles, which are visual, auditory, and kinesthetic. No matter what type of learner you are predominately, if you constantly use all three styles it helps to lock the information into your brain.

I have also noticed that these steps train you to have a photographic memory. This is especially important when there is a long chart you need to memorize. For example, in pediatric nursing you need to know a very extensive growth and development chart, and if you do not have kids yet it can be extremely foreign.

At first, incorporating this new study method may be challenging. But once you start using it and see your exam results rise, you will never turn back.

After you have looked over the words, pictures and highlighted sentences, then the next thing to do, of course, is go to class. While you are in class sit up straight in your chair and actively participate in the instructor's lecture. The most obvious way to do this is to take notes. You do not have to write down every word the professor says, in fact that will probably be impossible. But you do want to write down the main topics with a few supporting sentences at least.

When the professor says something you do not understand raise your hand and ask for clarification. I constantly asked questions during class. Some people would see me raise my hand, and I would hear a big sigh out of them. The majority of the people, though, came up to me after class and thanked me for asking questions because they benefited from further clarification. The thing is you have plenty of information to study already, and in class professors go over main points. For your exams, however, you need to know the subject in much greater detail.

Therefore, if you know what material the instructor is presenting in class you are already that much ahead of the game. You can now focus on the next items in the topic. I will give you an example of this: You are in class and the instructor is describing congestive heart failure. Your professor will go over introductory information such as the age of onset, the typical group of people who suffer from this disease, the drugs that can help, and the typical signs and symptoms. Usually they only have time to mention the main topics which can be found in the book. Remember though, as a general rule your questions will not be straight from the book. A sample question on the subject given above could be focused on educating the patient about possible medications and the therapeutic/negative side effects. This answer may or may not be word-for-word from your textbook or class discussions. But it is information you need to know.

Remember this as well – if you have a question, probably about one-third of the class has the same question. You will probably notice that when you ask the question your classmates will respond and say things like, "yeah, I didn't understand that either." You are all very smart to be in nursing school. From my personal experience, I would venture to say that 75% of the people who start out in nursing change their majors because it is too difficult. Also, material in nursing school is far from common sense. This is hard information to learn, especially if you have no medical background.

It is also good to remember that you are paying for your education. It is the instructor's responsibility to help you go to the next level. This level includes passing your classes and ultimately the NCLEX examination. It is their job to help you understand the material. So remember that when the words coming out of the instructor's mouth start to sound like a foreign language, do whatever it takes to get his/her attention and then ask for clarification.

Of course you do need to be mindful of your classmates and make sure you do not tie up too much of the professor's time during class. Like I said before, there is so much material that needs to be covered there is simply not enough class time. I found it helpful to always have a piece of paper handy designated for questions only. As soon as the instructor started speaking the different language I would jot down the word as best I could and then approach the instructor either after class or in a private session. Jotting it down helped me trust that I would eventually understand the material and thus enabled me to move on and focus on the next topics.

Do not have anything planned for immediately after class. Give yourself at least 30 minutes. Many nursing professors have so much information to impart that the classes often go longer than expected. Keep in mind how much material nursing encompasses. Make sure you do not plan anything immediately afterward so you can be available if the instructor is giving you more information. After the instructor has finished remain in your seat and look over everything -- all the bold words, pictures, and highlighted sentences. This time include the notes you just took. This process should not take longer than 15 minutes.

Sometimes after the class the teacher gets bombarded by a flood of students. In this case, I asked another student if he or she understood the areas where I needed clarification. I was always amazed how different subjects were crystal clear to others and were simply gibberish to me. But the same concept worked in reverse. At times, I was able to help my classmates when they were confused. How we can all listen to the same lecture and understand different things still baffles me today. But that is exactly what happens in a classroom.

The next tip to get the most out of your classroom experience is to sit near positive people. Many of us underestimate how much negativity can cripple us. The way I would find out if someone is positive or not is to first observe the person. Negative people typically are easy to spot by their body language, posture, and the words they speak. Initially, I would avoid individuals who portrayed a slumped posture and unfriendly facial expressions.

On the other hand there are tons of negative people who do not show their attitude so obviously. The way I would discover a person's true attitude would be to ask simple questions. Take for example, someone complaining about the cost of gas. I would say something positive like, "Yes, it is expensive, but more than 92% of the world does not have a car." A truly positive person would take that statement to heart and say something along these lines, "Oh I guess I didn't look at it that way."

People who mainly portray negative attitudes, and who want to stay that way, will do anything to stay in that state. More often than not, this person would go to a completely different subject and start complaining all over again. If you do this exercise you will find that positive people will be drawn to you. Or as the law of attraction states, like attracts like. You will also notice that negative people will not want to be around you because you are not a comfort to them as they complain. Surrounding yourself with positive people will make your nursing school experience so much better. (This applies to life, in general, as well!) Honestly, nursing school is hard enough on its own. It is nice to have uplifting people around you to lend a nice word or two when you need it.

What if you do this test to all the students in your nursing class and every one of them is negative? Sit alone. Nursing school usually takes about two years of your life. This may seem like a long time in the beginning. But trust me, it flies by. Be sure you do not completely block out the people you have perceived to be negative for the entire length of nursing school. You'll find yourself in situations where you can ask questions again and see if their attitudes are different. We all can be negative in particular circumstances. The main point of this exercise is not to isolate you but to insure you find the fun and happy people who you really want to be around.

We are never promised another day. Because time may be short, it is even more important to surround ourselves with people who will help us be successful through their "can-do" and happy attitudes. This personal story by Gail Cardoso is a reminder of how precious our lives are and how, even though we try to use our time wisely, we are never promised another day.

Gail's Story

"I graduated from an Associate Degree program and am currently the manager of an operating room in a community hospital in Massachusetts. Since taking this job, I thought a lot about going back to school for my BSN I had five classes left to take when I decided to take a 'break' from school. It was only supposed to be one semester but then turned into 18 months off. In April of 2008, I was at work and fell and got a bleed in my brain. I was rushed into Brigham Women's hospital and had emergency surgery within four hours. I was fine in the recovery room and later when I was moved to a neurologic ICU. To make a long story short, I bled the next day and again was rushed in for emergency surgery. This surgery was more involved than the one the day before. They ended up taking part of my cranium due to the significant bleeding that occurred.

"I was in a medically induced coma for almost two weeks, and then slowly regained consciousness. To say it was trying for my family is an understatement. I then was released to a rehab facility for physical therapy. Once getting home, I was still in a fog and at a loss as to what I would do with the rest of my life. I am one of those people who received a lot of my identity from being a nurse. My biggest fear was that I could never get back into nursing. While I was recuperating I looked at myself and wondered how I had let taking off 'just one' semester grow into almost two years away from completing my degree. Everyone was telling me I was being too hard on myself etc., etc. I chose to reenroll in the fall of 2008; I knew that if I could complete my BSN then I could still be a nurse.

"I took three classes that semester and slowly found my way back into nursing. For me, this degree is not just about getting the three letters after my name. It really saved my life. I will graduate on May 9, 2009, with the knowledge that even though it is just three letters, it helped me to find myself again. I had forgotten how much I need challenges in my life. It has also greatly impacted my nursing career. I now know how much more having the undergraduate degree under my belt has opened doors for me both personally and professionally.

"I definitely treat my patients differently now than I did two years ago. I can be much more empathetic, and it is because of getting my degree. The first part of my nursing career was all about memorization of signs and symptoms, medications and much more, as we all know. This degree encompasses so much more than that. It has made me look much deeper into things, and always to try to go that one step further. If anyone had told me that I would someday go to grad school, I would not have believed them, but here I am pondering the idea.

"My accident has made me realize my whole life should be a journey, and to make the absolute most of it whenever the opportunity arises. When I remember my accident, I thank God everyday for putting those nurses in my life to care for me. I now know firsthand that when taking care of patients they have given me the greatest gift of all, and that in itself is the privilege and ultimate trust that is bestowed on a nurse."

Gail Cardoso, RN
Emmanuel College

Chapter 6

How to Make the Best Use of Your
FREE TIME

I love the increased knowledge of medical diagnosis and procedures. There is always something new to learn. Also, the money isn't bad either!

Susan Poe, RN

Nurse for 24 years

Specialty: geriatrics

Now let me attempt to read your mind, you are thinking, "What free time? I have to wake up at 5 in the morning to get the kids up, dressed, fed, and to school. Then I go to school myself, and when I'm done, I have to go pick up the kids, feed them again, take them to ballet, soccer, and spend some quality time with them. Then once they are with the baby sitter I must go to work so I can pay my car payment, rent, and utilities. After all that, my significant other comes home and wants to spend time with ME. What free time are you talking about?"

I know those of you who do not have kids see different scenarios than the one presented above. But basically, you were still alarmed that I would assume you have an abundance of this luxury called "time." But that is exactly what I do think. The average American watches television. I don't care how much you watch, if you watch any, then, you watch television. Tell me how television is going to help you get a good grade on your next nursing school exam? Believe it or not learning how to holler "STAT" like that hunk or babe on *Grey's Anatomy* isn't going to help, honest.

I am confident when I say that the television is not going to add one point to your nursing school exam. Also, you can be sure you will not see anything of that sort on the NCLEX examination. So if I were you, I would cut out TV completely. I would even be cautious in watching the news, because it can keep you intrigued and glued to the screen by telling you things you "must" know. But think about it. At least for now, do you really need to know that information? Maybe about some subjects, and in this case, watch the one event and then turn it off immediately. When I started nursing school I completely cut out the TV and now that I have graduated and am working, I don't see any reason to go back. In fact, not watching TV gave me the time to write this book for you!

But the time I am really talking about is the time you spend doing the monotonous things. The things you do every day and could probably do in your sleep if you had to. These include brushing your teeth, driving to school or work, sweeping the floor, dusting the house, cleaning your car, all of the things that do not demand your full attention. Basically, these activities do not use a lot of brain cells. Which is precisely why I say you have free time! Your brain, in other words, has free time, and you could use that time to exercise it and learn something new to help you succeed.

The way you do this is you get NCLEX review CDs or DVDs, which you can find anywhere. I personally used ATI, which stands for Assessment Technologies Institute, LLC. What I absolutely loved about these DVDs was how they clearly broke everything down into easy-to-find sections. This is important because nursing itself is broken down into four or five major parts. I say four or five because some of the associate degree programs do not include community health as a section.

These DVDs are divided into sections like your classes in nursing school, so that for whatever class you are taking at the time there is a correlating DVD you can use to study and learn. Let's say you are in medical surgical nursing. You can take that DVD and play it while you're doing your habitual driving. Of course, you must use your auditory learning at this time and focus on driving safely. At first, I used my laptop, but it didn't seem loud enough. It also became beat up from the wear and tear of being used in the car so much.

My mother surprised me with a DVD player for my birthday, and it worked perfectly. DVD players are made specifically for travel, and normally are much louder than computers because they are designed to watch movies. Also, the DVD players are so much cheaper in relation to actual laptops, making them more affordable. While you're driving you simply listen to your lecture instead of the radio! Of course, you could always tape record your lectures, which is also a good idea. I would still encourage you to get the DVDs because hearing and visualizing things said in different ways is always beneficial. Also, my DVD's sound quality is so much clearer than tape or mp3 recorded lectures.

How to Succeed in Nursing School

So while you're driving, brushing your teeth, combing your hair, cooking dinner, cleaning the house, and not watching television(!), you can turn these on and have your own private instructor who you can start and stop whenever you need to! And if that is not cool enough, you can actually use this method even when you are surrounded by people. For example, if you're waiting at the doctor's office, riding the metro, or studying in the library, you simply plug in a pair of head phones and "voila," your private teaching session has begun!

You may say that after going to school all day and following your daily routine, you simply cannot pay attention. What I found was that when this happened, I would just let my mind wander to wherever it needed to be. Eventually, something from the DVD would catch my attention and bring me back. Even though you are not actively listening you're still learning. Remember the exercise I shared with you about just looking at the word before class? There you are using your visual field to familiarize yourself to the material and here you are using your auditory senses.

Listening to audios even if you are not paying 100% attention can have a major impact on how well you learn the topic. Your subconscious mind is still hearing what is being said and works at familiarizing itself with the information even when you are not consciously doing so! In nursing school, one of the biggest classes or sections is called medical surgical nursing. This class presents numerous different diseases. The DVDs do the same thing although they do not present as many diseases. They focus on the major ones. Discussion on each disease is about 15 to 30 minutes long depending on the complexity. The majority of the time you will have about four to eight of these topics on a test, and you could easily listen to these over and over.

What you will notice is that after you have listened to these sections over and over, even if you were not actively listening, eventually you will be "zoned in" and ready to learn the material to a very high degree. The reason for this is because you have heard these words several times and you will realize after hearing them repeatedly that they must be important. Once you zone in and learn what the DVD is teaching, you will have a much greater understanding of that section.

Also, as you read your textbooks you will notice that a lot of the material repeats itself, therefore making the reading much easier. It is very important though that you do this in addition to your reading. Although the DVDs go over the highly important topics, they do not encompass all of the information you truly need to know. What I believe they really do is take the biggest portion of the subject and break it down in ways that are easily understandable. That way you can focus on other things while you are reading.

If you haven't thought about it already, this would be a great thing to do prior to your lectures because, once again, if this is your second or third time to hear information, it will be much easier to retain. You would have to find out which topics were going to be discussed ahead of time, and then you could watch and listen to them ASAP. Imagine how successful you would be if you looked over the chapters in the book several times, watched the lecture on the DVDs, and finally went to class to solidify what you have learned! And these steps don't demand too much more time. They just teach you how to maximize the time you do have.

So what do these DVDs really offer? Well, first they cover the majority of the topics that you will be tested on in nursing school and on the NCLEX. These programs are precisely designed to prepare you to take the NCLEX. Many people I know didn't start studying for the NCLEX until after they graduated. You might still be successful if you wait until then, but things would be so much easier if your preparation starts earlier. Programs like these are an extremely good way to get a head start.

Each DVD program varies in the informational content. I will give you a brief review of what I have seen them contain. They usually start with a review of the anatomy and physiology. This is a very brief section, touching on the imperative information under the assumption that you didn't forget everything you learned prior to nursing school. After that brief review they talk about diseases, including the drugs used to treat each disease.

They usually mention if there are dangerous side effects to the medication and they also say what foods, drinks, or other drugs a patient should avoid while on the therapy. Remember that patient education is extremely important, so you want to be sure you pay close attention. Most of the programs also have books that coincide with the DVDs. The books offer a more detailed explanation of the disease process. They also offer any graphs or tables of information that need to be memorized, and most of them also offer NCLEX type questions.

After discussing disease-related information, the DVDs usually give you an example scenario. For instance, a patient comes to the hospital saying he is having difficulty breathing. Upon admission the patient's vital signs are: blood pressure = 146/89, respirations = 36 per minute, temperature = 97.7, heart rate 110, and oxygen saturation level is 84 %. What would you be most concerned about? Often, this scenario will be on screen with actors playing the patient and nurse. Then they would tell you the answer is oxygen saturation!

Furthermore, these DVDs teach valuable memory tools. For example, an acronym for a patient who is dehydrated would be, the higher the dryer. What that means is that the levels of electrolytes in your blood may appear higher if you are dehydrated because they are concentrated. But the beauty of the memory tricks is that they are a concept which could work with any patient in this condition. I have to tell you that these memory tools helped me on the NCLEX tremendously.

So where do you find these resources? And the important information, how much money are we talking about? The Assessment Technologies Institute or ATI can be found at: www.atitesting.com. The complete package cost $429. But before you get choked up at spending that kind of money, think about how much you already put into your education and how important it is for you to be successful as a student and on the NCLEX. The information offered in these DVDs is invaluable and definitely worth the money. Of course, there are many options available to you. Keep in mind that you may also be able to find these programs secondhand on eBay for much less. Another consideration is to split the cost with a classmate that you study with regularly.

As a final tip, I'll mention using flashcards, which some students find helpful. I believe they are less effective for nursing school than other methods I've discussed. You need to be careful about what you're going to put on the flashcards because there is so much information that you could be making flashcards 24/7 and never have time to review them. So my advice to you is to study the material at least three times first using the looking over method, attending lectures, and then watching the DVDs. Then, if necessary, you could make flashcards for material you do not understand.

Caroline Porter Thomas

Chapter 7

10 Steps to Effective Studying

Even a bad day in nursing is better than a good day at the other jobs I've had.

Sandy C. Muse, RN

Nurse for 25 years

Specialty: med-surg

Imagine you are sitting down trying to study. Your course load reading is over six chapters and your exam is in a week. How do you learn all of the required material? Where do you even begin? Now is the time to think "critically." But what does this word actually mean, and more importantly, how can you do it? Almost all of my nursing instructors asked us what critical thinking meant to us. The students' answers would vary with the usual, "thinking about thinking," "being actively thinking," or "carefully making decisions." But no one ever described how it was actually done.

Since this is a word I constantly heard, I developed a study method around it. This system helped me graduate with honors and pass the NCLEX examination the first time, completing only 75 questions, which is the minimum needed to pass. You may ask how I developed this study method and will it work for you? Well, I am by no means a gifted student. In fact, far from it. In the eighth grade I was held back and tested for learning disabilities. When I was in high school, I had to repeat several classes over the summer. I did manage to somehow complete a dual enrollment program my senior year thanks to grade forgiveness and my mother's constant help with tutoring. By the time I graduated high school, I was sure I would never enter another classroom again.

But as the story goes, I found myself right back between the dreaded walls, years later in college. But this time it was different. I was paying for it! So in order to avoid losing a ton of money, I had to pass. Little by little I started experimenting because common methods of studying were not working for me. I certainly needed to be more engaged in the material and started discovering how I could accomplish this. As I developed my study methodology, my grades started going from C's to A's. I started receiving invitations to join the honors club and I now hungrily sought material that I previously viewed as impossible. My techniques also helped me gain acceptance into nursing school.

I soon discovered however, that the same steps that helped me succeed in college were not good enough for upper division nursing classes. Changes in my study habits had to occur in order for me to successfully complete my nurse training. At first, this was very frustrating. I had no idea how to do it. Then, I started experimenting once again and made a few powerful additions to my study method that finally allowed me to thrive in nursing school!

I want you to use your study time most effectively, so it may be time to change your previous study techniques. This process is what really helped me take my grades in nursing school from C's to A's. I believe that if you follow my suggestions closely, and do everything listed, you will be successful on any nursing test you take.

Without any further delay, here are the steps:

"CRITICALLY!"

1. **Clear your mind first and set a schedule.**

2. **Review NCLEX questions.**

3. **Immerse yourself in the reading.**

4. **Test your knowledge.**

5. **Interact with your classmates and study together.**

6. **Contact your instructor.**

7. **Allow plenty of time for sleep.**

8. **Lecture Someone Else.**

9. **Learn to refocus your attention.**

10. **Don't forget Yourself.**

Clear Your Mind First and Set a Schedule

Just so you know, a few of these may be common sense. But what I've noticed about myself and others is that common sense is not always common practice. I want you to keep this list handy, referring to it often so you can remember these steps and use them daily. The initial step is to, **Clear your mind first and set a schedule.** This basically means writing down your agenda and thoughts. Leonardo da Vinci attributed his success to this one simple habit. He quickly jotted down his goals and ideas as they came to him. If this worked for Leonardo, then it can help you be successful in nursing school.

Scheduling should be done several times each day, beginning the night before and continuing at additional times the next day. Prioritize your assignments, exams, and projects. The idea is to open your eyes every morning and know exactly what your goals are for the day. I recommend planning your schedule in a journal just before going to sleep, maybe even while sitting on your bed. This first schedule is a general template of what you will be doing the next day. Say, for instance, you have class from 8 to 12. You can schedule your study block from 2 to 6. Once you have finished, leave your journal right there next to you so that if you forget to write something down you can easily add it later. This will help you sleep better because you will go to sleep with a clear mind, knowing that your list will be waiting for you upon awakening.

In addition, a mid-day scheduling should be done to evaluate your productivity and determine if there is anything else you can do to take full advantage of the day. This is extremely simple and can be incorporated into your day no matter how busy you are. Ask yourself, "What can I do to make sure my studying is effective?" Don't worry if nothing comes to mind immediately. In fact, you will probably find that when you initially ask the question, this will be the case. Surprisingly, you may notice that when you are not thinking about it, the perfect answer will dart into your mind. This is why it is important to have the journal close by so you can relax, knowing your keys to effective learning are safely written down. Some things that may come to mind are: If I study at the library, I will be more effective because there will be fewer distractions. Or if I go to bed earlier, I will be able to study in the morning more effectively because I will be rested. Realize that each day brings different circumstances and events, so you must ask this question every single day.

A final scheduling should be done right before you begin your study session. This needs to be a written, detailed agenda using every minute you allotted from the night before. If you think it is easy to sit down for four hours straight and be able to pay complete and total attention to a subject, I think you'll find it may be more challenging than expected. Soon enough, you may find your thoughts drifting off and, if you're not careful, you could lose hours of study time just by not using your time wisely. One of the best things you can do is to divide up the study session. Breaking up your assignments into separate sections makes it seem a lot easier than tackling a huge assignment as a whole. What you want to do is create your study session like a fun race and your opponent is the clock!

Let's say you scheduled a four-hour block to study. You may have a group presentation in your nursing fundamental's class that you need to research. Also, in two days you have a medical-surgical (med-surg) exam. And finally, next week you have an exam for community health. Prioritizing is the key when you have limited time. The most important thing to study for right now is the med-surg exam because that is coming up the soonest. So I recommend beginning and ending your study session with this topic, then incorporating the other assignments in the middle. Allow only two minutes to organize and write down your study session. Also, use words that will make you laugh or make you feel motivated to keep going fast! For example, my list might say:

- Med-Surg – 2 to 2:55

- Bathroom Break… hurry, the clock is ticking!

- Quick, find a great research article for Nursing Fundamentals on "Hand washing" 3 to 3:30.

- Back to Med-Surg, 3:30 to 4:30! Exam in 2 days! I MUST KNOW THIS!

- Now spend 1 hour studying for Community Health 4:30 to 5:30… GO!

- Finally, wrap up Med-surg 5:30 to 6:00.

- Whoooo Hoooooo! I'M DONE!

Review NCLEX Questions

Now that you have made your schedule, it's time to actually study. We will begin with the second step which is to **Review NCLEX questions** on the subject you are studying. You may think this step is improperly placed because traditionally we read a section and then test our knowledge by answering questions. However, if you review NCLEX questions first, you will stimulate your brain. Even though you probably won't know the answers, you will be exposed to the most important topics in that particular subject. This step will also familiarize you to NCLEX type questions. And while reading later, you will say to yourself, "Oh, that's why that question is right."

The NCLEX review books have a section of questions followed by the answer and rationales. Most of the NCLEX books I've seen even gave the rationale for the reasons why the wrong choices were incorrect. When you read the questions, you may be able to answer some correctly with the knowledge you have gained from previous sections. The main thing that is important is that you simply read everything. This includes the question, all the choices, and all of the answers and rationales. Do this fast, 15-20 minutes max, and don't worry about understanding everything.

So where do you get these questions? I used *Mosby's Reviews and Rationales*. But there are several NCLEX review books out there that are absolutely great. Other books are Saunders, Drexel, and Lippincott's. The NCLEX review book used while you are in nursing school is different than the one you use after you have graduated and are only studying for the NCLEX. The type of review book you need while attending school should be separated into four or five subject areas. These main sections are medical-surgical, pediatrics, psychiatric, obstetrics, and sometimes a fifth topic called community health.

The next thing you want to look for is that each main section is again broken down into smaller sections. For example, medical-surgical has sections labeled cardiovascular, respiratory and so forth. This is important because not every book does this. Many books just have a series of NCLEX type tests with a certain number of questions covering all subject matter in random order. This type of NCLEX review book will be most helpful for you after you graduate and are solely studying for boards. I suggest you check amazon.com or ebay.com to see if you can purchase slightly used books cheaply.

Immerse Yourself in the Reading

So now you are ready to completely and totally **Immerse yourself in the reading.** The way you accomplish this is by actively interacting with the material while you are reading. I would write in my book, read out loud, and underline every sentence that seemed important, sometimes underlining entire pages! This does make resale harder, but I think I got all that money back with my first nursing paycheck! You can also try standing up while you study to change things up a bit. Basically, experiment and see what works for you! When you write in your book, I highly recommend using a pencil and not a highlighter because when I read a page that has already been highlighted, I tend to only go toward those words. This may cause you to miss important information. Since you can erase pencil and not highlighter, I found using a pencil allows more flexibility when rereading a section.

Another way to keep yourself immersed in the reading is to keep a computer right in front of you with Google and dictionary.com open and ready to be used. In addition, any reference material, such as a medical dictionary or drug resource book, would be useful. As you read, pay special attention to the words you do not understand. How can you understand a paragraph if you do not understand all the words? So as soon as you come across a word you don't know, look it up. Immediately write the meaning down in the book with your pencil.

Also, whenever you are reading about a procedure, add visuals to enhance your understanding of the concepts. Your textbooks generally offer tons of pictures and these are great. Pay special attention to them. But also, if you are reading about something that does not have a picture, you can always search for the procedure in Google and see if you can get information there. This will help you learn by using more of your senses, which assists you in understanding and remembering the material.

Test Your Knowledge

Now, to complete your daily personal study session you must, **Test your knowledge** for about 20-30 minutes with questions. Again? Yes, again. And I may even say AGAIN! I believe this statement to be 100% true: The probability of you passing the NCLEX examination and your nursing school exams is directly proportional to the number of questions you complete. For me, it wasn't until halfway through my first year of nursing school that I understood the power of reviewing NCLEX questions. But once I figured this out, I persistently answered question after question. By the time I graduated I completed over 5,000 questions. This sounds like a lot, but if you consistently answer questions, it will not significantly lengthen your daily study time.

The difference between the initial review of NCLEX questions (step 2 Review) and this step is that you are now trying to apply what you have just read. The first questions you want to do are the same NCLEX questions you did to start your study session. You want to repeat these to make sure you understand the concepts that were presented before you move on. After you have done that, answer the study questions in your course book. Finally, practice NCLEX questions on a computer. Since the NCLEX exam is given on a computer, it is beneficial to acclimate yourself to this testing format.

When I first started nursing school, I was actually intimidated by questions presented on a computer. Initially, I had a difficult time reading on a computer and would print out everything possible so I didn't have to stare at the screen. Well, the only way to get used to answering questions on a computer is to do question after question. In just a short time you will notice how much easier it is to read and answer questions on screen. Most textbooks and NCLEX review books come with companion CDs that contain additional questions to complete on the computer.

Interact with you Classmates and Study Together

Once you have done all of these steps on your own, I encourage you to participate in an **Interactive group study** session with other motivated classmates. Sometimes, if you start the group study sessions when none of you know anything about the subject, the session can turn into social hour. Being a nursing student does not allow much time for leisure activities, so it is important to use your time wisely. Making sure you have sufficient knowledge of the topic is a great advantage when you collaborate in your group study sessions.

Studying with other smart individuals is an absolutely great way to get the knowledge hardwired into your brain. Remember, while you study together, different things are going to stand out for each member of the group. Some concepts will be easier for you to understand than it will be for others and vice versa. So, if you are studying with your group and you come across something you do not understand, take the time to ask your classmates so they can assist you. Have them do the same for you as well.

I assure you that group study sessions work as long as each member stays focused. Many times while testing a vision of my friend describing a concept would pop into my mind as I read a question. It was as if someone was giving me the answers to the test and all I had to do was listen. Working together is a great way to help everyone achieve success, but you must also be careful about whom you choose to work with. There are people who can make group study detrimental to you and others, and they should be avoided. I also highly encourage limiting your study group to no more than five students who are committed to helping each other. Also, keep in mind that group study is not for everyone. If you feel like you can accomplish more on your own than with a group, I would encourage you to work alone.

Contact Your Instructor

After you have done your best to understand the material, the next step is to "**Contact your instructors**" referencing any areas you do not understand. Go straight to the source and ask questions of the one who is going to test you on the material and give you a grade. Become close to your instructors since most instructors are very nice and will go out of their way to help you understand the material. Generally, the objective of most instructors is to impart their knowledge to you. Another reason to approach your instructors is to point out the specific areas you do not understand. Sometimes instructors noticed that there were many students asking about a particular topic. Consequently, they arranged extra sessions for large groups so everyone could go over the material with them.

I have to admit that some instructors do seem unapproachable at first. Don't let that stop you. Some instructors put on a hard front in the beginning so students will not try to take advantage of them. What happened a few times to me was that during the first week of class I labeled an instructor as approachable or unapproachable, caring or uncaring. Usually, I was wrong about my initial judgment and was surprised on several occasions by the willingness of the instructor to provide extra help or clarification. Another interesting observation was that the instructors who gave off an unapproachable aura seemed to have more time to help because they were not being bombarded by other students. The opposite was also true; nice and approachable instructors were constantly bombarded by students and hardly ever seemed to have time. So the bottom line is approach the unapproachable whenever necessary!

Allow Plenty of Time for Sleep

"Allowing plenty of time for sleep" is the next step. Have you ever studied so hard and were so stressed out about a test that you literally stayed up all night? How did you do on that test? You probably did not do as well as you could have. It is frustrating to later review the questions and realize you actually knew the right answers. You simply marked the wrong one by mistake or you read the question wrong. Whatever the reason, your mind cannot function at optimal capacity unless all of its needs have been met. And one of those needs is the need for sleep.

Marci Shimoff, in her book *Happy for No Reason,* described an interesting study that presented data supporting the idea that sleeping has a greater impact on your happiness than your household income or marriage. So there is no doubt sleep is a vital human need. You also know from taking anatomy and physiology class that most healing that occurs in your body happens at night. When you schedule time for rest, your body will thank you by helping you in achieving your study goals.

Also, have you ever noticed how you can be thinking about a difficult concept, fall asleep thinking about it and then wake up knowing the answer? It is crystal clear to you because even though you were asleep, your subconscious is working hard to figure everything out. Try it sometime. Go to sleep when you have been studying for a long time and cannot grasp the information. You may be too tired to think about the topic. When you wake up notice how much easier the material is for you to understand. Another suggestion to ensure your body receives appropriate rest would be to go to bed earlier and plan a morning study session. Do whatever works for you, but just make sure you give your body the rest it needs.

Lecture Someone Else

Continuing on with the ten steps to effective studying, the first L stands for "**Lecture.**" Lecturing someone else is one of the best ways to ingrain knowledge in your mind. Have you ever possessed knowledge of something that you have not been able to teach someone else? If so, has it ever come to the point where you needed to look at something differently so you could teach yourself how to explain it to another? After you have explored the subject from a different angle, then taught it, you probably had a much deeper understanding of it!

Teaching someone else requires a thorough understanding about the subject and, while you teach another, your knowledge will increase exponentially. Not only that, but you will be helping those around you. So when you hear a classmate complain about not understanding something, this will be your opportunity to help. Don't worry, in nursing school there will be plenty such opportunities!

Learn to Refocus Your Attention

Learning to refocus your attention means learning to redirect your focus once your brain has started wandering. When you have been sitting down studying for a while, you may begin to feel tired and your ability to concentrate diminishes. Most people at this moment grab a cup of coffee or quit studying. However, there are many things you can do to get the exact same feeling as coffee that will allow you to refocus your mind and continue studying. I would drink a cup of hot water with lemon during my study sessions. Hot water alone gives you a good feeling that is similar to the feeling of coffee. The lemon just adds a nice flavor to it. Another technique I used to maintain my focus while studying was to listen to motivating music. Songs from inspirational movie soundtracks always seem to keep me on task.

Sometimes, a quick break is needed that can help make a long study session more productive. During my breaks, I would jump up and down, dance around, or bounce on a trampoline that I had one at home. This would really pump me up, enabling me to actively interact with the study material once I finished my break. In addition, while I was moving around, feeling good, and having fun, I would see myself studying with 100% attention focused on the subjects I wanted to learn. I would only need to get pumped up for about three to five minutes before I could not wait to get back into my chair so I could learn the material and ace the test. I would do this about every two hours or so. You may need to do it more or less depending on how well you are able to focus at the time. Of course, there are many other things you can do to help refocus your attention. You could do 20 jumping jacks, take a quick walk outside and get some fresh air, or take a power shower. These activities may improve blood circulation and reenergize you so that you can focus on studying.

Sometimes these techniques didn't work for me and I subsequently discovered that I needed to figure out why my mind was wandering. I realized there were three reasons that were usually the root cause. These were: 1.) I was worried or stressed about something 2.) I had been studying for too long and my body began to physically hurt; or 3.) I was completely bored. So once I discovered the root cause of my inability to focus I would try to do something about it. If I was worried or stressed about something, I would try to take immediate action to relieve the stress. Let's say I was stressed about another class besides the one I was studying for. I would take a break from what I was originally studying and then study fervently for the other class, allowing myself 30 minutes for this diversion. Once I did something toward improving in that class, I would feel much better and be able to refocus my attention on other areas.

Sometimes, I would be stressed out about things in my life I had little control over. Examples of these could be complicated family, money, or relationship issues. Unfortunately, thinking about these stressful issues was affecting my ability to study and learn. So I would do a mental exercise to help myself focus on what was important. Specifically, I would think about the subject that was stressing me, allowing myself to feel all the feelings that went along with it. Often, these were feelings that were painful and irresolvable. However, feeling pain can be very useful if you employ it correctly. Here is the key: After briefly feeling the pain, I would imagine I failed nursing school because of my inability to focus. With the pain being doubled and unbearable to think about, I would rethink about my issues and see if it was possible that I was looking at the worst-case scenario and not the actual facts. Many times, I was worried about things that were so far from happening that 95% of the time they never happened! As a result, I developed the faith that everything works out in my favor. This exercise always made me feel much stronger than before. Once I was able to refocus my energy, I was immediately able to continue my studying.

The second reason my mind wandered was from physical irritation. After studying about an hour or two in the same position, my back would start to hurt! At first without thinking, I would reach for an Ibuprofen or Tylenol and in about 30 minutes my pain would be gone. Then a few months later at Christmas, my brother bought me a Pilates ball. I fell in love with it because after I had been studying hard for awhile with every single muscle at full attention, I would just lie back on that ball and feel absolutely, wonderfully relaxed. Unfortunately, I have a dog that is notorious for destroying all kinds of things by biting into them and one day he took a big bite into my poor Pilates ball. But since my back felt so good from stretching like that, I decided that I did not need the ball. So I would lean over couches or big chairs, anything that would support my weight. It pretty much gives you the same feeling as the ball. Eventually, I started incorporating stretching into my study sessions. I found that a quick stretch every hour or two would help me concentrate for much longer periods of time.

The third situation that caused my mind to take a mental vacation was when I was completely bored with the topic. It was at times like this that I would try and take a step back, and think about why I was going through all of this hard work. One of my biggest dreams was to be the kind of nurse who made a real difference in the lives of my patients. I wanted them to feel the love that emanated from my hands as I touched them during my assessments. I also wanted to help my patients smile through the hard times and share a laugh with them. My passion is to serve my patients in every way possible. Then, I would remember the Chinese proverb, "A gem cannot be polished without friction" and I would see how this boring topic was the friction I needed to help me reach my dream.

Here is another tool which helped me through uninteresting topics. Since nursing school was so time consuming, I was unable to generate income. Consequently, there were many times that I didn't have everything I needed or wanted. In order to get over my studying block, I would imagine how great it would be when I was finished with nursing school, working in a hospital and finally making money! I looked at how much money I had then, which was somewhere in the negative range, and then would focus on all the money I would make as a nurse. Next, I would say to myself, "The only thing stopping me from getting there is a little test on a boring subject!" After all that, I definitely had the energy and power to get the necessary studying done. It is interesting how money, or lack thereof, can motivate us. And also remember, every component of your nursing education is needed so you can be the best nurse possible.

Don't Forget Yourself

The final step in the CRITICALLY mnemonic process is the **Y** that stands for "don't forget Yourself." This simply means that whenever you have done well in an area or have pushed yourself as hard as you possibly can, reward yourself. So many times we beat ourselves up when we do something we consider to be stupid or wrong. But we pay no attention when we do a good job. We may even find ourselves downplaying how well we did. Maybe you studied hard for a test, got a great grade, and then told yourself that the test was not that hard to begin with. If you find yourself doing this, take the time to look yourself in the eye with a mirror and say, "Good job, you earned this, that was excellent." You deserve the positive feedback!

I would like to finish this chapter with a quote from the great Albert Einstein. "Genius is 1% inspiration and 99% perspiration." In this chapter, I have shared with you all of the shortcuts and techniques that helped me. I wish I could take the tests for you, or at least give you an A for your effort, but it's not possible. So apply what you have learned and never give up. Remember that each day will bring you closer and closer to your dream of being a nurse. Use your days wisely!

Caroline Porter Thomas

Chapter 8

Mastering NCLEX Questions

I decided to become a nurse in the first grade and I have stuck to my decision. What I love best about being a nurse is helping people and teaching each one about something they need to know about themselves and medicine. If I had to make a new decision today, I would choose nursing. It has both its rewarding and bad days, but it only takes one thank you and that makes it all worth it.

Sue S. Copelan, RN

Nurse for 42 year

Specialty: emergency department

So how do you take what you have just learned from studying with the CRITICALLY mnemonic and apply it to test questions? Unfortunately, as I mentioned in earlier chapters, nursing questions are rarely simply knowledge based. What that means is you will almost never see a question that is directly from your reading material. More likely you will have a patient, sometimes called client, who is experiencing a disease and you need to know what nursing responsibilities are important to do and in what order.

These questions represent real-life scenarios that you could experience as a nurse. The challenge, of course, is that you're not a nurse yet, and yet you need to think as if you were already a nurse. As many of my instructors said, the NCLEX is not made for nursing students, it is made for nurses. Because of the detail and vast amount of information you need to know, it is very difficult to commit the information to memory. Not only that, each question is extremely difficult to read, and misinterpreting one of the words in the question will probably cost you the entire question. Then when you finally understand what is being asked, you must choose the best choice from four right answers.

If we put this scenario into everyday life, we understand why the nursing questions are difficult and complex. A patient does not come to you and say, "Hey, I'm suffering from irritable bowel syndrome." The patient comes to you with prolonged diarrhea, painful stomach cramps, and unexplained weight loss. Also, one patient can be suffering from many different things, so understanding which problem needs to be addressed first is important. For example, a burn victim is suffering from disturbed body image and also fluid balance overload. You must understand that although the disturbed body image is important, the fluid balance overload could potentially be fatal if not cared for immediately.

The NCLEX is based on one basic principle. That is, will the test taker be "safe" while practicing nursing? The questions, though they seem impossible at first, are really designed to make you think and be observant to every detail. The goal for every student nurse should be, of course, to succeed in passing the NCLEX, and become knowledgeable enough to practice "safe nursing."

You can pass the NCLEX in 75 questions; imagine two to four years of schooling being validated with 75 questions. You may ask how someone could determine if you are a competent nurse from just 75 questions. The answer is because in order to answer each question you need to know four to five different concepts. In essence, you are really answering about 375 questions. Most nursing instructors are going to model their test questions in the same way the NCLEX does so you are familiar with these types of questions.

It is a great advantage for you to know the character of typical nursing test questions before you take your first exam. I remember failing my first nursing test! It was the first test I had failed in two years! It did not have one definition, matching, or fill in the blank question; it consisted solely of scenario questions. I am sure my instructor warned us and tried to prepare us, but I definitely did not grasp what she was saying. Then, after the test, I and many other students spent about two hours griping and complaining about how the test didn't cover what we studied.

So how do you read, understand, and correctly answer nursing questions? The first thing is you must learn how to read the question. You must read every single question as carefully as you would if it was a real-life event and involved someone you deeply cared about. That means actively reading the question to the highest degree. We are at a slight disadvantage in the classroom because in our testing centers we cannot use all of our senses like we can when we are alone. If we read the question out loud we will get kicked out of the class room.

In the classroom, the first thing to do is to read the question three different times. It may seem you do not need to do that, especially with the easy questions. I said the same thing; I would even think to myself that I do not have enough time to read the questions three times. However, when I kept reading the questions too fast and making simple mistakes that cost me good grades, I changed my mind. Typically, we read a question and an answer pops in our heads, usually the most obvious one. Regardless, you need to take a step back and reread the question. After you have reread the question, look at all of the possible choices and, if you are unable to find another possible answer, then go with your first instinct.

This method works well, but it is still important to practice reading questions before you even get the test. Review NCLEX questions in a review book and read the questions out loud. Listen to yourself as you read the questions. The reason for this is because we can think and read much faster than we can speak. Verbalizing the questions out loud will develop a good pace in your mind for when you read the questions on a test.

The next component of answering the questions is obviously choosing the right answer. When you study on your own with NCLEX questions, cover up the choices and think about what the answers could be. Try to remember what you have learned about the topic. Write down any thoughts that come to your mind. After you read the question at least two times you can see the choices and see if any of them were similar to what you were thinking.

The next thing to do is to compare answer choices. Often, you will not understand the question so the choices are a great way to get clues. If you read them carefully, more often than not, you have two answers that are similar. Once you establish the similarities, you can see which are the distracters, the similar ones, or the different ones. You must be careful, though, because distracters often seem like the obvious answer if the question is read wrong. That is why it is important to read the question three times before making your final selection.

A tip that I found helpful for the NCLEX was that some choices suggest things that as a nurse you would never do. These choices would not be obvious for the lay person. For example, if a patient is taking a psychiatric medication that is known to harm an unborn baby (teratogenic) and the patient is trying to get pregnant, then an obvious answer would be to tell the patient to discontinue the drug beforehand . If you were to choose this answer, even though the patient would need to discontinue the drug, you would be wrong.

This is because you need to discontinue psychiatric medications slowly under a doctor's supervision because abrupt discontinuation could have fatal consequences. This rule applies to almost all medications; doctor's supervision is important. So looking for why an answer could be wrong is a good way to eventually get to the right choice by the process of elimination. Choices such as those make the process a little easier by immediately eliminating choices.

Another good way to choose the answer is to always think, if this were to happen what would kill or cause catastrophic harm to this patient first? Soon, if you have not already, you will learn about the ABCs and this stands for airway, breathing and circulation. Interference with any one of these three processes presents an immediate threat to life. Without even one of these, a human being will die or lose an extremity in a matter of minutes. This is looking at the worst-case scenario and then planning your care in order to prevent it from happening.

Take, for example, a patient who was in a car accident and has multiple injuries. They may have broken ribs and leg bones, but they are also having difficulty breathing. The most important thing for you to do is to help this person's breathing. Only then can you treat other issues. In nursing school, this knowledge will help you, especially in the beginning. As time goes by and the questions get more difficult, you will see fewer of them related to the ABCs. To be a safe nurse you must recognize the potential for these problems, and take actions as deemed necessary to prevent crisis. When patients become critical, there are normally many signs and symptoms hours or even days before it happens. Recognizing these signs early on not only saves the patient from traumatic rescue methods, like intubation and mechanical ventilation, but may save his/her life.

I like this personal journey story from Bryne Martin because she shares some of the tips she learned in nursing school – and offers much-needed words of encouragement.

How to Succeed in Nursing School

Bryne Martin's Story

"In my last semester of nursing school, in the midst of taking finals and studying for the NCLEX, I found myself reflecting on the past four semesters. There were many good times and many bad times, stressful weeks that seemed never ending, and way more studying than I ever thought possible. There are numerous lessons and tricks I learned that helped me to get through difficult tests and will help me when I finally become an RN.

Hot and dry, sugar's high; cold and clammy, need some candy.

"There is a professor at my school who is known for her exceptional knowledge of the human body, as well as the exceptional difficulty of her class. While my classmates and I spent two hours every Thursday and Friday morning frantically taking notes and wondering how in the world we could learn all of this material for a test, she lectured on and on about diabetes and hypertension, obesity and seizures. Though I cannot remember every detail and occasionally find myself having to review notes from her class, there are some things I will not forget. She always had some saying, no matter how corny, that seemed to really stick and always seemed to be my saving grace on a test. For diabetes, it was 'hot and dry, sugar's high; cold and clammy, need some candy.' In treating heart attacks, remember, 'MONA (morphine, oxygen, nitroglycerine, aspirin) greets all patients!' When studying, come up with your own sayings to simplify material and make it easier to remember. We all laughed at the time, but to this day, those sayings were the most helpful tidbits I learned in any class.

The greatest test is the test of life!

"The teacher with all the sayings had one in particular that was obviously her favorite. She was always telling us that while it is important to know all the material for her tests, the test that really mattered was the test of life. Again, we laughed, because honestly, her tests were more than difficult, and she wanted us to worry about the test of life! But she was right. Though my friends and I are still students for a little longer, some of us have encountered our first life tests. There have been patients who tried to die on our watch, and that is the time when what you know really matters. You cannot go back and study your notes when a patient is pulling a respiration rate of 6 breaths per minute or suddenly has a blood pressure of 68/45. It all comes down to what you know. Don't just learn to pass the test next week. Learn it and really take it in because when it all comes down to your practice and you are not a student any longer, you'll be taking the greatest test -- the test of life.

Patients are people too

"The pediatric rotation is usually the most fun because your patients are cute kids, and sometimes, you get to just play with them. Take note when you step onto a pediatric floor and you'll see bright colors and toys, but be sure to really see the nurses. They have a particular joy in their work. Their patients have taught them that sickness does not always mean sadness. Kids are resilient, and though they are sick, they are still kids. They want to have fun and laugh. Patients are not their disease; they are people. While adult units do not have the rainbows and colors and light that pediatric units have, a patient is a patient, no matter how old or young. Laugh with your patients. Ask them about their lives outside of the hospital. See that they are people and treat them as such. Once you realize that sickness does not always mean sadness, you will find a true joy in helping people through a difficult time.

From classmate to friend

"The interesting thing about college, and especially nursing school, is that there are so many people at different stages of life. In my nursing class of 82 students, there are seven who are married, four with kids, and a few who are engaged. There is a girl from Pakistan, a few who already have a degree, no men, two going into the military right after graduation, and so many other interesting characteristics that make our group what it is. The single girls admire the ones who are married because it must be difficult to manage a husband while doing all of the work of nursing school. The married girls admire the ones with kids because, while a husband can sometimes be like a child, how do you study with a baby crying? There's always something interesting about classmates.

"Over the past two years, we have suffered together, been grossed out and saddened and frustrated together. We have grown together. Now, with graduation in sight, we still celebrate together and count down together. Get to know your nursing classmates. They will laugh at your stories and understand your frustrations better than anyone else could. They can help you to understand electrolyte imbalances, will always be there for study sessions and a good laugh, and they will become true friends. You may move away and never see them again or you may end up working in the same hospital for years to come. No matter what, you will always have inside jokes and late-night cram sessions.

Nursing is the most respected profession in the United States

"Many instructors consider nursing to be the most respected profession in the United States. When I first heard this, I had my doubts because one might think people would have more respect for doctors or religious leaders, not nurses. Looking at my experiences over the past two years, I'm beginning to really believe nurses might be the most respected professionals. The pay is not always great. Our duties are not always appealing or attractive. It takes a special person to be a nurse, though.

"There are quite disgusting things we see and do, and having the stomach to handle those events is not something that comes easily to some people. While we do not have the power doctors have, nursing school is nothing short of difficult. We are expected to know the anatomy and physiology of the human body, many disease processes, medications and their effects, different lab tests and their normal values, interventions, nursing care, nursing theory, community resources, and alternative therapies.

"A day of work includes, but is not limited to, caring for multiple patients, administering medications, retrieving vitals and performing assessments, consulting with doctors, working with staff of different disciplines (physical therapy, diabetes educators, dieticians, etc.), assisting patients with hygiene and physical therapy, and charting all tasks performed. We spend a lot of time teaching our patients about everything from diet to medications, disease processes to discharge care. We are nurses, or at least, we will be soon! This is something to be proud of, and I am. Of all the lessons I've learned in nursing school, I think this is by far the most important."

Bryne Martin, BSN, RN

The University of Texas at Austin

Chapter 9

Advice for Papers, Presentations, Pharmacology and Clinical

Nursing is hard and can try your patience, but in the end when you can send a patient home, knowing it was with your help that they could even go home, you realize it was worth it.

Angie Hinkle, LPN

Nurse for 1 year

Specialty: med-surg

Now I'm sure many of you will not jump for joy when you get your research paper assignment. You probably reluctantly did them in the past, reading tons of books, journals, and magazines. You had to find research from multiple sources, and then type an excessively long paper about topics that were of absolutely no interest to you. You lost sleep, time, fun, and tons of things you wanted to do all because of the dreaded research paper. I know because I've been there.

I found a way to make research papers a lot easier. Most of the time in nursing school you will use nursing journals for the data. Try to always start out with three to five journals and find about five interesting facts or sentences from each. The best way to find the journals is to use a site that has access to medical/nursing journals. You cannot find this information on Google. Most of the published authors want you to either buy their journal or buy access to a website that posts their journals. Most schools, however, give you access to certain web sites where you can find the journals free of charge (or, should I say, for the small price you are paying for your college education). But to save you research time on Google, look first at the site your school offers. Either your instructor or the librarian can help you find this.

Once you have read and gathered adequate knowledge and sentences from the research, begin thinking about what your paper is going to entail and create an outline of the main topics. Under each of the main topics, put as many quotes as you can. Try to do this in an order that would make sense. If you need to, you can put the quotes first and organize later. Then as you are writing your paper, simply follow the outline. Sometimes it took me an entire week to get the outline the way I wanted it. But when the outline is strong, the paper will just flow. And the paper that took me an entire week to plan is oftentimes written in a few hours.

Another thing that I wanted to share with you that made my nursing school life a little easier was Reference Point Software. This is a program that you can simply install on your computer and it formats your word document to APA (American Psychological Association) style. This format is commonly used for writing papers and citing sources in scientific professions, and is used by most nursing schools. It is quite a bit different from the MLA format you are probably used to.

Formatting your paper to APA guidelines is quite complex and could take a lot of time to learn. Small, thick books with very small print words are available for purchase if you want. After reading the entire book you will be able to follow the directions by reading each step and putting your paper in the right format. Or you can purchase the software for about $25, which is probably the same price as the book and it does everything for you. You decide.

It's not that I'm lazy, and I don't think for one second that you are. I know you could get that APA book and do it yourself. The question is why? In nursing school you will have much to do, and you need to learn how to organize your time better than you ever had to before. So why not make life a little easier? Reference Point Software made APA format a breeze. I used to get stressed out because I had no clue where to even start when it came to formatting the document. After getting the program, I was able to focus on the content of the document.

So let me describe how to use this software. Install the program following the on-screen directions. The CD will show you a short video that walks you through how to use the software. When you start writing a paper, the software works in conjunction with Microsoft Word. On the toolbar at the top of Word, you will notice a section that says APA. You click on that and it will start asking you a few questions, for example, "What is the title of your paper," "type your name," and so on and so forth. Then it will say, "Are you ready to start the body?" Click yes, and start typing the paper.

Once you have completed the body of the paper, you are ready to document your citations. Simply click on the word references at the top. A list will scroll down asking whether the source is a book, journal, magazine, or from online; choose the appropriate source. This was my favorite part of the entire program because correct citation can be an absolute pain with all of the periods, semicolons, and words that need to be capitalized. All you have to do is answer the questions. The program directs you to type in the title of the source, then the year it was written, and then the author's name. It does everything for you. Life is so easy sometimes!

The software is available at www.ReferencePointSoftware.com. If you have written a paper in the APA or MLA style you know how valuable a program like this is. You will save hours of headache and hard work. You will be able to focus on the meat of your paper instead of the little details. Work smarter, not harder!

Another thing you are going to need resources for is group projects. Before I started nursing school, I didn't like group projects. When I finished I decided I could live the rest of my life without doing another one again. I'm not exactly sure why our professors insist we do these, but I think it is because as nurses, we have to work together. I have personally witnessed this working in the profession. For many things we do, another nurse must witness that you have done what you said. Also there are many tasks that cannot be carried out by one nurse, so you need to help each other to accomplish everything that needs to be done.

Regardless of why, team projects will be a big part of your nursing school so you need to prepare yourself. For my group projects, I always wanted to present something that no one else would do, something that was creative and would impress others. The only problem was that when you do these projects, you must have adequate resources to back them up. Normally you use research findings from journals like the ones mentioned before. Be sure you choose a topic that has a good amount of information already written about it. Unfortunately, many of my creative and exciting ideas did not have much available.

Before you decide on your topic, do this. Put the subject you are researching in your journal research engine. If you do not find at least three or four journals related to this topic, change your search terminology. Your entire presentation or group paper is basically going to be about the data that was found in your resources; if you cannot find data, then you have no information for your project. Some of the topics with plenty of research were hand washing, turning patients who cannot turn themselves every two hours, and the "Five Rights" when administering drugs.

Pharmacology

One of the most difficult portions of nursing school is pharmacology. There are thousands of different drugs, and you should be knowledgeable about the ones you will be administering. You need to know the generic and name brand, its mechanism of action, therapeutic benefits, side effects and much more. Pharmacology is probably the most confusing part of nursing school because it requires learning a huge amount of information. Then instead of knowledge-based questions you must utilize the information to answer scenario questions.

I recommend using the *Prentice Hall Nurse's Drug Guide* as your drug book, because this is the company that writes the NCLEX questions. This book, as the title suggests, is completely geared toward nurses. Most drug books try to accommodate everyone in the healthcare industry including pharmacists, doctors, and last but never least, nurses! What happens if there are tons of sections that we as nurses do not understand? Then the reference will not have all the information we need to know to be safe practicing nurses.

Another resource I recommend is a book called *Pharmacology Made Insanely Easy!* by Loretta Manning and Sylvia Rayfield. I didn't come in contact with this book until after I graduated and Ms. Manning came to my school to do an NCLEX review. I struggled with pharmacology the entire time I was in nursing school. In three days with Ms. Manning and using the tools and techniques presented in this wonderful book, I learned more about drugs than I did in two years!

In their book, Ms. Manning and Ms. Rayfield presented the drugs in the form of classes. Instead of looking at each drug individually, tackling thousands upon thousands of drugs, you focus on a much smaller number of classes of drugs. The benefit of looking at drugs in this way is that you can determine a lot of information about the drug, even when you have never heard of that exact one before! The book includes tons of pictures and then short explanations about the pictures and how it helps you remember the drug information.

This book is heaven sent for the visual learner, but it also includes many songs created to tunes we all know. For example, they take the title "Three Amino Mice." These three mice represent the negative side effects of the class of drugs called aminoglycosides. Then they created catchy drug information phrases to be sung to the tune of "Three Blind Mice." This type of learning taps into the right side or creative side of your brain, which helps you learn and retain the information easily. I recommend you get this book ASAP and use it along with your pharmacology and drug book.

Clinical

Clinical is by far the most important part of nursing school. This teaches you by example instead of by theory. Sometimes you will be paired up with an excellent nurse, while other times you're not so lucky. Use each experience wisely and learn from everything. When I was paired with a competent, positive nurse, I would learn by example. When paired up with the opposite, I learned what not to do.

Always bring your textbooks to clinical. There may be times when you do not have much to do. Use this time to look up your patient's diagnosis, medications, and to work on your care plan. You can find a wealth of information in the patient's chart. Read the history, which tells a lot about what kind of person the patient is and explains why he or she is in the hospital. Spend time with your patient. When was the last time he/she had a bath or had their hair washed? Do they need anything? Many times, they may just need someone to talk to.

This may be a difficult time for many of you. This is when you may see seriously ill patients and it can be extremely overwhelming and emotional. Amanda Miller has been a nurse for three years. This next story was written when she was in nursing school as a journal entry.

Amanda's Story

"So the last three weeks have been a test for me. What exactly I am being tested on I'm not sure. But I have a sense of peace today. Maybe it is because this is the first day I've been able to rest. Maybe it's because I survived my first CCU clinical without completely breaking down.

"I have beefs with God. I have never claimed to be a devotedly religious person. I have come to believe a few things through trial and error though. Nursing school has definitely pushed me. I've fought it, and blamed my parents; I've threatened to quit numerous times. I've drunk myself stupid on occasion because I didn't know how to deal with what I was feeling. I have been scared to the point of tears. I have been anxious to the point that sweat poured down my back. I have been stupid in front of my peers. I have been brilliant in front of my instructors. I have struggled through it all.

"The other day, I was sitting outside in the hallway studying for a test that proved to be impossible. A classmate, whom I rarely talked to, had been on a trip to India to volunteer in an impoverished town to offer medical attention to their children. I had stumbled across her pictures on Facebook and admired her bravery for going so far away to someplace with so little. So I told her that. She just smiled, meekly, and said, 'It was hard to go there, but it was hard to leave too.' She told me it was really a different world over there. Then she said something that I hope will stick with me, she said 'God gives us grace at the moment we need it most, and not a minute too soon.'

"Monday, I had to go pick up my patient from the hospital (for you who haven't a clue: that means I got permission to sit in a back room and review a chart before I took on my patient the next day). I got what I needed. I went to ask my nurse what to expect and my anxiety level shot through the roof. My guy was on a ventilator; he was very, very, very sick. Lines and tubes, everywhere. I knew the settings on the vent, I knew the lines and tubes. But actually seeing all of it come out of one, withered, dying man… just hurt me. I started crying. I do not think quickly on my feet. I do not like to be put in situations where people's lives are truly my responsibility. But I had to for clinical.

"I had to do it for nursing school, and that scared the crap out of me! My nurse was exceptional. She walked me through everything; she calmed me down so I could actually retain what she had to say. She mothered me until I was okay with it. Then I went home and called my instructor. I cried to her about how this man scared me. I called my momma and squalled to her about it. I cried to Chelsea and David about it after that. I was sincerely horrified about this man. He couldn't talk to me. He couldn't respond to me. He had nine different IV lines, a tube feeding, a vent, and he didn't know I was there… I had done a lot of worrying and crying over this man since 2:30 that afternoon. By 9:30, I was mentally stripped of any rational thought. I was asleep by 9:31.

"Five o'clock came really early. I didn't think about the patient while I got ready. I ate my cereal. I picked my friend Chrissy up and we rode to the hospital together. I was fine while I got report. I walked through his door and started crying again. All the different drugs had him sedated while a machine breathed for him. But his eyes were open. He didn't see me through the haze… but his eyes were open. I touched his hand, and let my tears fall on his bed, I told him I was scared. I told him I wasn't cut out for this. I told him I didn't have any idea what I was supposed to do. I know none of this registered to him. I know he will never know I was there – or that I bathed him, rubbed lotion on him, massaged his arms and legs, turned him, brushed his teeth, shaved his face, or that I had come to the reality that sometimes, admitting our worst fear out loud, even if on deaf ears, helps us move forward, helps us find strength. I realized then that God gave me grace when I needed it, but not a minute to soon – just so he could watch me grow."

Caroline Porter Thomas

Chapter 10

Advice from Nursing Professors Nationwide

Nursing has allowed me to become a good person and also provided for my family.

Chris Burns, RN

Nurse for 23 years

Specialty: emergency department

"Nursing Professors Care"

Maria Carpenter, *RN, MSN*

Professor, Highline Community College

"Nursing instructors really want students to succeed. I went into teaching because I enjoy studying, and that moment of 'Aha! I get it!' when that mental light bulb would suddenly turn on. I wanted to share that with students. Even when material is difficult, I believe there is a way to reach that moment of understanding. The challenge is how. What learning strategies can help? What can I, as an instructor, do differently? Nursing instructors like students. I enjoy and welcome students visiting me in my office or sending me emails. While we nursing instructors cannot take the test for you, or write that report for you, we can and want to work with you.

"We have knowledge about resources: not just books, but people who may be able to help you. I have students come to me struggling with personal issues that are interfering with their focus on their studies. Some even question whether they should drop out. I can offer them resources for counseling -- including our own college counseling center, which offers services free of charge. Many colleges have this service. When faced with personal stressors or crisis, counseling can have a huge impact on promoting well-being in all facets of one's life.

"Communicate with your instructors! is one recommendation I emphasize. If I know a student is missing classes because of extenuating circumstances (e.g. illness), I am empathetic and very willing to help out as much as I can. Likewise, if a student is struggling, but makes the effort to come see me, I recognize the student sincerely wants to succeed, and enthusiastically offer what I can. I don't chase down no-show students to ensure they have all the handouts, lecture notes, etc. they need. I don't chase down students that are at risk for failing. I assume they are adult learners.

"Instructors appreciate feedback -- both positive and negative. It helps us 'keep our fingers on the pulse' of the class. (I do not wait until the end of the course for students to evaluate me and my teaching -- I have students do an evaluation midway through the course as well). Naturally we like to know what is going well. But equally, if not more important, we like to know what is not going well."

Advice from Professors Nationwide

Jane Brokel, *PhD, RN*

Assistant Professor, University of Iowa

1. **What do you think it takes to be successful in nursing school?**

    "Commitment to the profession with long-term learning."

2. **What do you think students should do to prepare themselves before they start nursing school?**

    "Develop reading and studying skills."

3. **What is your view on the amount of material that is covered in nursing school?**

    "The amount is not the issue but learning a process to manage and use information with evidence is more important... information literacy."

4. **What do you think is the most common avoidable mistake students make in nursing school?**

    "Not reading and using the data, information and knowledge obtained from reading."

5. **How often do the most successful students visit you for extra help?**

    "At least once but most keep close contact"

6.   **Approximately how many hours would you predict the average successful student studies daily for their nursing classes?**

"5 hours or more."

7.   **What is the biggest contributor that you feel helped students pass the NCLEX examination?**

"Skills of critical thinking and reasoning; using several of your learning styles, eg. group activities, interactive."

8.   **Do you think most students need a formal NCLEX review to prepare for the exam?**

"Yes"

9.   **What are some basic things that you see the successful students doing on a daily basis?**

"Attendance, reads all materials, studies regularly, prepared for class and clinical assignments, participation in team/group activities both in classroom and outside classroom as related to being engaged in your new profession."

Georgia Anderson, *MSN, RN*

Professor, Salt Lake Community College

1.   **What do you think it takes to be successful in nursing school?**

"Desire to learn, support from employers and family, willingness to invest time, good ethical compass, study buddies, good reading and writing skills."

2.   **What do you think students should do to prepare themselves before they start nursing school?**

"Have a computer, high speed internet, healthcare insurance, some money in savings."

3. **What is your view on the amount of material that is covered in nursing school?**

    "No doubt about it, there is a lot. It's necessary."

4. **What do you think is the most common avoidable mistake students make in nursing school?**

    "Cheating."

5. **How often do the most successful students visit you for extra help?**

    "The ones who need it often avoid me. The ones who don't visit often."

6. **Approximately how many hours would you predict the average successful student studies daily for their nursing classes?**

    "4-5 hours."

7. **What is the biggest contributor that you feel helped students pass the NCLEX examination?**

    "Studying daily. Not just for the NCLEX but for the courses."

8. **Do you think most students need a formal NCLEX review to prepare for the exam?**

    "No."

9. **What are some basic things that you see the successful students doing on a daily basis?**

    "Reviewing readings daily, studying in groups with other successful students, reviewing class notes daily, making school their first priority, asking questions."

10. **Do you have any motivational statements or quotes you have created that you would like to pass on to nursing students?**

"You are of above average intelligence. If you weren't, you wouldn't be here. Don't ever let your behavior suggest otherwise."

Nancy Baumhover, *RN, MSN, CCRN*

Clinical Assistant Professor, Arizona State University

1. **What do you think it takes to be successful in nursing school?**

"Motivation, passion, communication, critical thinking, and confidence."

2. **What do you think students should do to prepare themselves before they start nursing school?**

"Examine how well they've performed in the sciences previously. Gain better study skills and exposure (work in a hospital)."

3. **What is your view on the amount of material that is covered in nursing school?**

"Curriculums are packed with material. Unfortunately, most of which is necessary to ensure the development of a knowledgeable and safe generalist clinicians."

4. **What do you think is the most common avoidable mistake students make in nursing school?**

"They do not read their text!"

5. **How often do the most successful students visit you for extra help?**

"The only visits I receive are for remediation."

6. Approximately how many hours would you predict the average successful student studies daily for their nursing classes?

"Unsure. Maybe ask some successful students"

7. What is the biggest contributor that you feel helped students pass the NCLEX examination?

"A sound curriculum, ATI testing and a NCLEX preparation course."

8. Do you think most students need a formal NCLEX review to prepare for the exam?

"Yes. It certainly can't hurt."

9. What are some basic things that you see the successful students doing on a daily basis?

"Devise a plan and manage time to study, read text, understand personal learning style, limit other roles while in school (for example limit work or other responsibility), and maintain a 'healthy' amount of anxiety."

Mary Brann *MSN, RN*

Assistant Professor, Touro University

1. What do you think it takes to be successful in nursing school?

"Determination, dedication, time to do work outside of class, social support."

2. What do you think students should do to prepare themselves before they start nursing school?

"Study basic math calculations and word problems; work on basic medical terminology; visit someone in the hospital; interview an RN".

3. **What is your view on the amount of material that is covered in nursing school?**

    "By necessity, there is a lot of material. It is the job of the instructor to sort through it for the essentials (and after that there is still a lot!)

4. **What do you think is the most common avoidable mistake students make in nursing school?**

    "Not taking it seriously; arriving late; not using all the academic resources available to them."

5. **How often do the most successful students visit you for extra help?**

    "Not often."

6. **Approximately how many hours would you predict the average successful student studies daily for their nursing classes?**

    "3-6 hours."

7. **What is the biggest contributor that you feel helped students pass the NCLEX examination?**

    "Determination; self confidence; reviewing content and test taking skills."

8. **Do you think most students need a formal NCLEX review to prepare for the exam?**

    "I believe it builds their confidence, but they still need to study!"

9. **What are some basic things that you see the successful students doing on a daily basis?**

    "Coming to every class; attending extra remediation/review classes; studying; asking questions; offering to help others; seeking new experiences in clinical."

10. **Do you have any motivational statements or quotes you have created that you would like to pass on to nursing students?**

"Persevere!"

Elizabeth Campbell *PhD, MSN, FNP*

Professor, University of Alaska Anchorage

1. **What do you think it takes to be successful in nursing school?**

"Committed faculty, supportive administration."

2. **What do you think students should do to prepare themselves before they start nursing school?**

"Develop good study skills."

3. **What is your view on the amount of material that is covered in nursing school?**

"Adequate"

4. **What do you think is the most common avoidable mistake students make in nursing school?**

"Underestimate the rigor of nursing programs/not prepared for the amount of work."

5. **How often do the most successful students visit you for extra help?**

"Rarely"

6. **Approximately how many hours would you predict the average successful student studies daily for their nursing classes?**

"3-4 hours."

7.   **What is the biggest contributor that you feel helped students pass the NCLEX examination?**

"Consistently good school work performance."

8.   **Do you think most students need a formal NCLEX review to prepare for the exam?**

"No."

9.   **What are some basic things that you see the successful students doing on a daily basis?**

"School is a priority. They committed to putting the time in."

10.   **Do you have any motivational statements or quotes you have created that you would like to pass on to nursing students?**

"Think of the worst nurse you've ever seen. If he/she can become a nurse, you can too."

Dr. Sarina Roche *DNSc, MSN, RNC*

Nursing Department Chair,

Eastern Maine Community College

1.   **What do you think it takes to be successful in nursing school?**

"Study science skills, motivation and hard work."

2.   **What do you think students should do to prepare themselves before they start nursing school?**

"Learn terminology and have hospital experience."

3.   **What is your view on the amount of material that is covered in nursing school?**

"Lots, and progressively more difficult."

4. **What do you think is the most common avoidable mistake students make in nursing school?**

    "Not asking for help when struggling."

5. **How often do the most successful students visit you for extra help?**

    "As needed."

6. **Approximately how many hours would you predict the average successful student studies daily for their nursing classes?**

    "6 hours."

7. **What is the biggest contributor that you feel helped students pass the NCLEX examination?**

    "Practice questions."

8. **Do you think most students need a formal NCLEX review to prepare for the exam?**

    "Depends on how well they do in nursing school."

9. **What are some basic things that you see the successful students doing on a daily basis?**

    "Reading before class, studying daily, using a study group after class, review exams, working on test taking strategies with instructors."

10. **Do you have any motivational statements or quotes you have created that you would like to pass on to nursing students?**

    "Nursing is a great career. All the hard work is worth it!"

How to Succeed in Nursing School

Jean Auffarth, *PhD, MSN, RNC*

Professor, Southern Illinois University Edwardsville

1. **What do you think it takes to be successful in nursing school?**

   "Study time. Commitment to being a nurse."

2. **What do you think students should do to prepare themselves before they start nursing school?**

   "Realistic view of time involved (clinical). Need to understand all course information from past courses must be retained and used."

3. **What is your view on the amount of material that is covered in nursing school?**

   "Too much content."

4. **What do you think is the most common avoidable mistake students make in nursing school?**

   "Work too much and don't keep up with readings."

5. **How often do the most successful students visit you for extra help?**

   "Rarely."

6. **Approximately how many hours would you predict the average successful student studies daily for their nursing classes?**

   "4 hours."

7. **What is the biggest contributor that you feel helped students pass the NCLEX examination?**

   "Students with A's & B's. Cognitive ability to take tests"

8. **Do you think most students need a formal NCLEX review to prepare for the exam?**

"Yes."

9. **What are some basic things that you see the successful students doing on a daily basis?**

"Reading to understand material. Form study group. Keep up with class."

10. **Do you have any motivational statements or quotes you have created that you would like to pass on to nursing students?**

"Don't look back. Today is the path to the rest of your life."

Linda Pellico, *MSN, PhD, RN*

Assistant Professor, Yale University

1. **What do you think it takes to be successful in nursing school?**

"A supportive environment where skilled educators and clinicians can respond to students' questions/concerns. And clearly a bright, thoughtful student."

2. **What do you think students should do to prepare themselves before they start nursing school?**

"Spend time focusing on anatomy and physiology. If grounded in "normal" it will be easier to make connections with pathology."

3. **What is your view on the amount of material that is covered in nursing school?**

"Vast content range but it is incumbent upon educators to define core content and build on it as the program progresses. It is impossible to cover all content for nursing but crucial that we focus on core."

4.   **What do you think is the most common avoidable mistake students make in nursing school?**

"Assuming it will be easy."

5.   **How often do the most successful students visit you for extra help?**

"Not often. They are concerned about their peers that are less successful and aware that extra help is limited"

6.   **Approximately how many hours would you predict the average successful student studies daily for their nursing classes?**

"Three hours."

7.   **What is the biggest contributor that you feel helped students pass the NCLEX examination?**

"Testing students on high level items rather than simple or moderate levels. Adding exam items for each class given on blackboard. Completing 3,000 or more questions before taking the NCLEX".

8.   **Do you think most students need a formal NCLEX review to prepare for the exam?**

"No."

9.   **What are some basic things that you see the successful students doing on a daily basis?**

"Reviewing content before class, reviewing notes after class, taking prep questions on classes or on Blackboard, working in groups discussing the content, staying on top of content, not taking a week off from studying."

10.   **Do you have any motivational statements or quotes you have created that you would like to pass on to nursing students?**

"Not really. It's more an attitude and core belief that they can and will be successful rather than a cliché."

Caroline Porter Thomas

JoAnn Howell, *RN, BSN, MSN*

Instructor, Hutchinson Community College

1. **What do you think it takes to be successful in nursing school?**

    "Deep desire and determination."

2. **What do you think students should do to prepare themselves before they start nursing school?**

    "Review math skills – become a CNA."

3. **What is your view on the amount of material that is covered in nursing school?**

    "Overwhelming."

4. **What do you think is the most common avoidable mistake students make in nursing school?**

    "Procrastination."

5. **How often do the most successful students visit you for extra help?**

    "Very little – usually they are self motivated and listen well."

6. **Approximately how many hours would you predict the average successful student studies daily for their nursing classes?**

    "2-3 hours or more."

7. **What is the biggest contributor that you feel helped students pass the NCLEX examination?**

    "ATI testing (Assessment Technologies Institute)."

8. **Do you think most students need a formal NCLEX review to prepare for the exam?**

    "Yes."

9. **What are some basic things that you see the successful students doing on a daily basis?**

"Attending class, asking questions to clarify assignments, setting aside 2-3 hours/day to study, handing assignments in on time, working in study groups outside of class."

Anonymous

1. **What do you think it takes to be successful in nursing school?**

"Drive, a strong academic foundation and ability to increase and adapt critical thinking skills"

2. **What do you think students should do to prepare themselves before they start nursing school?**

"Work involving interaction with people and thinking on their feet. This work does not have to be directly related to healthcare, although it is helpful"

3. **What is your view on the amount of material that is covered in nursing school?**

"Mostly appropriate."

4. **What do you think is the most common avoidable mistake students make in nursing school?**

"Not addressing time management issues, 'getting by' in some classes."

5. **How often do the most successful students visit you for extra help?**

"About 80-90% of them visit."

6. **Approximately how many hours would you predict the average successful student studies daily for their nursing classes?**

" I am not sure."

7. **What is the biggest contributor that you feel helped students pass the NCLEX examination?**

"Strong test-taking skill development and practice."

8. **Do you think most students need a formal NCLEX review to prepare for the exam?**

"Yes."

9. **What are some basic things that you see the successful students doing on a daily basis?**

"Following up on resources and suggested activity by professors, active listening and/or participation in class work, keeping time; due date, etc. up to date, being accountable for their learning."

Jason E. Farley, *PhD, MPH, CRNP*

Professor, Johns Hopkins University

1. **What do you think it takes to be successful in nursing school?**

"An ability to synthesize didactic lecture and clinical experience to improve critical thinking."

2. **What do you think students should do to prepare themselves before they start nursing school?**

"Excellent understanding of basic anatomy and physiology."

3. **What is your view on the amount of material that is covered in nursing school?**

"The material is very broad and attempts to cover too many subjects. I think there should be more emphasis on inpatient medical-surgical skills and outpatient case management skills."

4. **What do you think is the most common avoidable mistake students make in nursing school?**

"Overconfidence."

5.   **How often do the most successful students visit you for extra help?**

"Occasionally."

6.   **Approximately how many hours would you predict the average successful student studies daily for their nursing classes?**

"2 hours for every 1 hour in class."

7.   **What is the biggest contributor that you feel helped students pass the NCLEX examination?**

"Paying attention in class (i.e. Not checking email, texting, talking). 2. Studying as noted in number 6."

8.   **Do you think most students need a formal NCLEX review to prepare for the exam?**

"Yes."

9.   **What are some basic things that you see the successful students doing on a daily basis?**

1. *"Come to clinical prepared. 2. Critical thinking practice on how to combine theory/practice.   3. Studying as in noted in number 6. 4. Group study sessions. 5. Ask informed questions."*

Nancy Winsor, *RRT, RN, MSN*

Professor, Lamar Community College

1.   **What do you think it takes to be successful in nursing school?**

"Complete dedication! Really, one must be organized and disciplined to get through the courses and actively learn the concepts."

2.   **What do you think students should do to prepare themselves before they start nursing school?**

"Increase their reading comprehension skills. Take courses on how to critically read. Take a critical thinking course. Get personal matters organized."

3.   **What is your view on the amount of material that is covered in nursing school?**

"Of course there is too much material and not enough time."

4.   **What do you think is the most common avoidable mistake students make in nursing school?**

"Biggest mistake is not putting in the time needed for each class outside the classroom time."

5.   **How often do the most successful students visit you for extra help?**

"At least twice/month."

6.   **Approximately how many hours would you predict the average successful student studies daily for their nursing classes?**

"I think they do not set up a daily schedule."

7.   **What is the biggest contributor that you feel helped students pass the NCLEX examination?**

"Critically reading the chapters."

8.   **Do you think most students need a formal NCLEX review to prepare for the exam?**

"I'm not sure but it wouldn't hurt, so yes."

9.   **What are some basic things that you see the successful students doing on a daily basis?**

"Study everyday 1-2 hours/course minimum, take notes, create an effective study group with a facilitator, seek help, ask questions."

10. **Do you have any motivational statements or quotes you have created that you would like to pass on to nursing students?**

"To me nursing school is like a serious illness, as Norman Cousins wrote: The more serious the illness, the more important it is for you to fight back, mobilizing your resources – spiritual, emotional, intellectual, physical."

Laura Meloche, *MSN, RN*

Assistant Professor, University of Wyoming

1. **What do you think it takes to be successful in nursing school?**

"Success in nursing school takes hard work, dedication and a lot of studying. The student has to read, comprehend and apply the information."

2. **What do you think students should do to prepare themselves before they start nursing school?**

"Be very strong in math and sciences."

3. **What is your view on the amount of material that is covered in nursing school?**

"I feel there is a lot covered. But if we teach you how to critically think and problem solve you can figure out whatever the content is."

4. **What do you think is the most common avoidable mistake students make in nursing school?**

"Studying the way they did in high school or in the prerequisite courses."

5. **How often do the most successful students visit you for extra help?**

"Very frequently."

6. **Approximately how many hours would you predict the average successful student studies daily for their nursing classes?**

    " 3-4 hours plus."

7. **What is the biggest contributor that you feel helped students pass the NCLEX examination?**

    "Starting to test them with application questions from day one. Teaching them the way a nurse thinks."

8. **Do you think most students need a formal NCLEX review to prepare for the exam?**

    "For the weaker students, although it can give the average student confidence."

9. **What are some basic things that you see the successful students doing on a daily basis?**

    "Studying, reading their books, coming to class prepared, asking questions, making connections between theory and clinical."

10. **Do you have any motivational statements or quotes you have created that you would like to pass on to nursing students?**

    "Nursing is the best profession in the world!"

Mike Aldridge, *MSN, RN, CCRN, CNS*

Professor, University of Texas at Austin

1. **What do you think it takes to be successful in nursing school?**

    "Good understanding of science, determination, support (friends/family/instructor)."

2. **What do you think students should do to prepare themselves before they start nursing school?**

"Have a good background in the pre-requisite coursework, learn how to study, volunteer/work in a healthcare setting."

3. **What is your view on the amount of material that is covered in nursing school?**

"It is a lot of material in a relatively short time. Learning facts/basic information is something students can learn from a book, but applying that information is best done in clinical or group setting."

4. **What do you think is the most common avoidable mistake students make in nursing school?**

"Getting behind in a course, since getting caught up is difficult due to the fast pace and the volume of the material."

5. **How often do the most successful students visit you for extra help?**

"Not very often, actually. The most successful students seem to "get it." The students who visit me are those who are struggling, or who want to debate a test question they missed."

6. **Approximately how many hours would you predict the average successful student studies daily for their nursing classes?**

"This number varies considerably, but I would guess 3-6 hours/day."

7. **What is the biggest contributor that you feel helped students pass the NCLEX examination?**

"Regular attendance in lecture and going through many practice questions to learn testing styles/test taking tips."

8. **Do you think most students need a formal NCLEX review to prepare for the exam?**

   "No, but I think the reviews are beneficial to those who take them."

9. **What are some basic things that you see the successful students doing on a daily basis?**

   "Forming study groups; reading before class; studying daily; focusing on understanding the material rather than memorizing it; taking time to relax/take a break."

10. **Do you have any motivational statements or quotes you have created that you would like to pass on to nursing students?**

    "I like to remind my students that upon completing nursing school you know a little about everything, but not a lot about anything. You will learn details once you are done with school. It is our purpose to teach you the basics and get you to think like a nurse. You can teach anyone how to do a skill, but it is hard to teach people to think."

Helen Ahearn, *MSN, RN*

Assistant Professor, Emmanuel College

1. **What do you think it takes to be successful in nursing school?**

   "Have excellent one-on-one relationships with faculty, take study/test taking skills classes, attend school with small classes, attend an accredited school."

2. **What do you think students should do to prepare themselves before they start nursing school?**

   "Study hard. Learn to memorize well. Take 1-2 years of Latin as it is the basis of all medical terminology."

3. **What is your view on the amount of material that is covered in nursing school?**

    "It is just the basic amount. More is needed to be successful in practice."

4. **What do you think is the most common avoidable mistake students make in nursing school?**

    "Being unorganized."

5. **How often do the most successful students visit you for extra help?**

    "I teach in an RN to BSN program. Students e-mail me with questions several times per week. I almost always stay after class for questions."

6. **Approximately how many hours would you predict the average successful student studies daily for their nursing classes?**

    "Several hours."

7. **What is the biggest contributor that you feel helped students pass the NCLEX examination?**

    "Take the preparation courses. Practicing daily as many questions as possible."

8. **Do you think most students need a formal NCLEX review to prepare for the exam?**

    "Yes."

9. **What are some basic things that you see the successful students doing on a daily basis?**

    "Plan ahead, know when assignments are due, review assignments, ask questions if the assignments are unclear, do all the reading, memorize what is needed to."

10. **Do you have any motivational statements or quotes you have created that you would like to pass on to nursing students?**

"Don't put off tomorrow what can be done today!" Thomas Jefferson

Dr. Susan Hayden, *RN, PHD*

Professor, Troy University

1. **What do you think it takes to be successful in nursing school?**

"Determination, desire and hard work as well as a real desire to be a nurse."

2. **What do you think students should do to prepare themselves before they start nursing school?**

"Work at least 6 months as a nursing assistant on a medical-surgical unit or in a nursing home."

3. **What is your view on the amount of material that is covered in nursing school?**

"Though it is massive, it is necessary."

4. **What do you think is the most common avoidable mistake students make in nursing school?**

"Ask for help too late."

5. **How often do the most successful students visit you for extra help?**

"The strong ones don't need to see me unless they have a specific problem. The weak ones, more than once a week."

6. **Approximately how many hours would you predict the average successful student studies daily for their nursing classes?**

5 hours over and above classes (2 hours for every hour spent in class the next day is ideal).

7. **What is the biggest contributor that you feel helped students pass the NCLEX examination?**

"Studying"

8. **Do you think most students need a formal NCLEX review to prepare for the exam?**

"Usually, the reviews are more about how to test-take than nursing knowledge i.e. stress reducing, how to think through a question."

9. **What are some basic things that you see the successful students doing on a daily basis?**

"Read, review, ask questions, attentively attend all classes, take care of themselves (diet, rest and exercise)."

10. **Do you have any motivational statements or quotes you have created that you would like to pass on to nursing students?**

Not my creation, but borrowed quotes;

"Can't never did."

"If you think you can't you won't."

"Teachers don't fail you – you fail yourself."

Caroline Porter Thomas

Michael Malay, *RN, MSN*

Professor, Western Nevada College

1. **What do you think it takes to be successful in nursing school?**

   "Read the book! Good study habits. Don't work full time during nursing school."

2. **What do you think students should do to prepare themselves before they start nursing school?**

   "Develop good study habits."

3. **What is your view on the amount of material that is covered in nursing school?**

   "Much greater than content in other degree areas."

4. **What do you think is the most common avoidable mistake students make in nursing school?**

   "Working too much while attending school."

5. **How often do the most successful students visit you for extra help?**

   "Infrequently."

6. **Approximately how many hours would you predict the average successful student studies daily for their nursing classes?**

   "2-3 hours"

7. **What is the biggest contributor that you feel helped students pass the NCLEX examination?**

   "Read the textbooks. Take an NCLEX review course."

8. **Do you think most students need a formal NCLEX review to prepare for the exam?**

   "No."

9. What are some basic things that you see the successful students doing on a daily basis?

"Read, review lectures, work on papers, study. Have no outside life."

Rita Antonson, *RN, MSN, APRN-NP*

Professor, University of Nebraska Medical College

1. What do you think it takes to be successful in nursing school?

"I think it's important for students to read all of the assigned readings, ask a lot of questions, and seek out new learning opportunities."

2. What do you think students should do to prepare themselves before they start nursing school?

"I believe it is important to take all of your prerequisites at a 4-year college to prepare you for the type of courses you take in nursing school."

3. What is your view on the amount of material that is covered in nursing school?

"I feel the material is adequate for baseline new nurse knowledge."

4. What do you think is the most common avoidable mistake students make in nursing school?

"I don't think they always spend enough time learning the information and instead memorize it for a test. This results in quick knowledge loss."

5. How often do the most successful students visit you for extra help?

"Rarely."

6. **Approximately how many hours would you predict the average successful student studies daily for their nursing classes?**

   "2 to 3 hours a day."

7. **What is the biggest contributor that you feel helped students pass the NCLEX examination?**

   "The amount of time and effort spent studying while in the program and taking an intensive review course in class proximately to NCLEX."

8. **Do you think most students need a formal NCLEX review to prepare for the exam?**

   "Yes. Absolutely, I would recommend it."

9. **What are some basic things that you see the successful students doing on a daily basis?**

   "Acting enthused to be in class or clinical, attempting problem solving, reading their textbooks, asking questions, not procrastinating."

Paula Oleson, *MSN, RN*

Program Director, South Texas College

1. **What do you think it takes to be successful in nursing school?**

   "Motivation, perseverance, family support, dedication to purpose."

2. **What do you think students should do to prepare themselves before they start nursing school?**

   "Take most difficult faculty, learn to learn, not memorize, learn how to use resources."

3.　　What is your view on the amount of material that is covered in nursing school?

"It is a lot, but only skims the surface of all that needs to be learned to be an excellent nurse not just a good nurse."

4.　　What do you think is the most common avoidable mistake students make in nursing school?

"Thinking it is easy. Not studying to learn. Not taking responsibility for previous material."

5.　　How often do the most successful students visit you for extra help?

"1-2 times a week."

6.　　Approximately how many hours would you predict the average successful student studies daily for their nursing classes?

"3-5 hours on average."

7.　　What is the biggest contributor that you feel helped students pass the NCLEX examination?

"Learning test taking strategies doing numerous test questions, developing testing stamina."

8.　　Do you think most students need a formal NCLEX review to prepare for the exam?

"Yes, they need to hear others rather than solely their own faculty give an overview."

9.　　What are some basic things that you see the successful students doing on a daily basis?

"Being on time, attending class, having a study group, reading material, reviewing exams, eating meals."

10. **Do you have any motivational statements or quotes you have created that you would like to pass on to nursing students?**

"Be the 'best' you can be!"

Maria Carpenter, *RN, MSN*

Professor, Highline Community College

1. **What do you think it takes to be successful in nursing school?**

"Commitment to studies, making nursing school a high priority, attending classes/clinical regularly."

2. **What do you think students should do to prepare themselves before they start nursing school?**

"First, have a plan for dealing with unexpected events (example: back-up for transportation, child care ect.) Secondly, elicit support from family, friends. Third is to Reduce life stressors as much as possible."

3. **What is your view on the amount of material that is covered in nursing school?**

"It is a substantial amount necessary to learn. Will likely continue to increase as nursing/healthcare becomes more complex."

4. **What do you think is the most common avoidable mistake students make in nursing school?**

"Too many activities outside nursing school. Working too many hours (>20 hours per week). Not studying on a regular basis, but cramming."

5. **How often do the most successful students visit you for extra help?**

Approximately 50% of them visit my office at least once per quarter.

6. **Approximately how many hours would you predict the average successful student studies daily for their nursing classes?**

   " 4-5 hours."

7. **What is the biggest contributor that you feel helped students pass the NCLEX examination?**

   "Having students self-study with comprehensive NCLEX-RN book concurrently with course/subject. This includes taking lots of NCLEX level practice questions."

8. **Do you think most students need a formal NCLEX review to prepare for the exam?**

   "No (but it does seem to increase their self-confidence)."

9. **What are some basic things that you see the successful students doing on a daily basis?**

   "Study independently and/or in a study group, get some type of physical exercise, check Blackboard postings, contribute to Blackboard discussions, ask for help, clarification of information as needed, and lastly, maintain a positive attitude."

10. **Do you have any motivational statements or quotes you have created that you would like to pass on to nursing students?**

    "Remind yourself how far you have already come. This is evidence that you have what it takes to keep going!"

   Regan Luken, *RN, MSN*

   Professor, University of South Dakota

1. **What do you think it takes to be successful in nursing school?**

   "Perseverance, focus, recognizing that nursing school takes top priority over social aspects, working in the healthcare

field in some capacity helps with certain concepts of safety, legal issues, basic patient care."

2. **What do you think students should do to prepare themselves before they start nursing school?**

    "Work in the healthcare field. Have a solid foundation in math, anatomy and physiology. Learn about critical thinking and how to answer application based questions versus black and white. Students can no longer rely solely on memorization of information."

3. **What is your view on the amount of material that is covered in nursing school?**

    "I teach for an ADN program which is 4 semesters. We have to cover a lot of material in a shorter period of time. The ideal curriculum is one that focuses on specific concepts (safety, aeration, ect.) rather than on separate topics."

4. **What do you think is the most common avoidable mistake students make in nursing school?**

    "They believe they can memorize everything from lecture and Power Points and fail to read their textbooks."

5. **How often do the most successful students visit you for extra help?**

    "Quite commonly because they are hungry for more information. They are motivated and it shows in their test scores."

6. **Approximately how many hours would you predict the average successful student studies daily for their nursing classes?**

    "3-4 hours."

7. **What is the biggest contributor that you feel helped students pass the NCLEX examination?**

    "Use of Kaplan program that includes study tools, exams through courses, remediation after exams, and NCLEX

review course. Also, from the beginning test students like the NCLEX will."

8. Do you think most students need a formal NCLEX review to prepare for the exam?

"Yes, definitely."

9. What are some basic things that you see the successful students doing on a daily basis?

"Reading, completing and reviewing online interactive case studies, studying, coming to class, taking their education seriously."

10. Do you have any motivational statements or quotes you have created that you would like to pass on to nursing students?

"Even the weakest student can become the strongest nurse by asking questions, and finding the answers. But most important is caring for and respecting their patients enough to go that extra mile."

Louis Bixby, *RN, BSN, MSN*

Beebe Medical Center

1. What do you think it takes to be successful in nursing school?

"To be passionate about nursing and to develop a sense of being eager to learn and to know."

2. What do you think students should do to prepare themselves before they start nursing school?

"Review A&P; discover their learning style, i.e. visual, auditory, kinesthetic; explore study skills that will work for them."

3. **What is your view on the amount of material that is covered in nursing school?**

   "It is a tremendous amount. The focus should be on "need to know" versus "nice to know."

4. **What do you think is the most common avoidable mistake students make in nursing school?**

   "Not following criteria for assignments, not being prepared. Preparation leads to enhancement of self-confidence."

5. **How often do the most successful students visit you for extra help?**

   "Not often. Usually it's the unsuccessful students who are trying to improve."

6. **Approximately how many hours would you predict the average successful student studies daily for their nursing classes?**

   No answer.

7. **What is the biggest contributor that you feel helped students pass the NCLEX examination?**

   "Review test taking skills by taking a review course, practicing computer programs, reviewing NCLEX questions, rest and relax the night before big exams."

8. **Do you think most students need a formal NCLEX review to prepare for the exam?**

   "Absolutely yes!"

9. **What are some basic things that you see the successful students doing on a daily basis?**

   "Review assignments and ask if they don't understand. They make sure to know what is expected the next day. Review notes or lessons of the day. Are prepared for clinical (assignments, diagnosis, A&P, uniform). Join a study group and find a role model. View criticism as useful."

10. **Do you have any motivational statements or quotes you have created that you would like to pass on to nursing students?**

"Take responsibility for yourself, nursing is an attitude and a commitment, make a choice to become socialized to the many roles of the nurse."

"The greatest glory in living lies not in ever falling, but in rising every time we fall."

– Ralph Waldo Emerson.

"People may fail many times, but they become failures only when they begin to blame someone else."

– Unknown.

"Have patience with all things, but first of all yourself."

– St. Frances De Sales

"If you scatter thorns don't go barefoot."

-Italian proverb

Caroline Porter Thomas

Chapter 11

How Do You Keep Going?

I love how I am able to make a difference as a nurse. I advise you to love your patients and consider them your children, at times scared and helpless. Make their journey to recovery easier by educating them, reassuring, and being there for them!

Tatiana Canton, RN

Nurse for 4 years

Specialty: critical care ICU,

trauma ICU and emergency department

Nursing school generally lasts between 1½-4 years, including prerequisites. Of course, such a range depends on which program you choose. So how do you keep going strong the entire time? When you first start, your attitude is something like, "Bring it on, I can handle anything!" Or at least that was my attitude. About a year into it, though, your juice just seems to run out and you find yourself praying for the day when it will all be over. You may find yourself not studying as hard as you used to. And you may even see some of your grades start to slip.

So when you notice yourself slipping, when you start to ignore the pile of books that even a heavyweight champion would have a hard time lifting -- stop right there. Simply ask yourself, what can I do right now to make myself feel better? What could I do that would really change my mood? The mood you are in determines the attitude you portray. If you are in a lazy mood and then something happened, say, for example, a child falls and hurts himself. What do you do? Do you sit there and say "I feel lazy, so the kid can wait, even if they are really hurt?" No! You get up and run over to the child and make sure they are ok.

You probably forgot that you felt lazy in the first place. You are just happy the child is okay. What you have done is established a new focus and that new focus was the safety of the child. If you can do it for the child, do you think you can do it for yourself? What if you could do something to put yourself in a constructive learning mood before you begin studying? If you are open minded and keep asking yourself what evokes that feeling for you, I promise you will indeed find something. Here are a few examples of the things that I did: bubble baths; daily time in prayer, meditation, exercise (especially stretching), relaxation, reflection time, writing in my journal, spending time communicating with friends, purchasing something I've been wanting for a while, and/or even sleeping.

When you take the time to make yourself feel better you will be surprised at how much more efficient you are when you study. Instead of spending 20 minutes on the first page trying to keep your eyes open, you will be able to relax knowing that you didn't neglect yourself. You will be able to study and, more importantly, retain what you study. Out of that list above, I absolutely loved to stretch. I constantly took about 20 to 30 minutes to just stretch. When I returned to the book I felt as if all the blood in my body had been circulated, refreshed, and re-oxygenated. Whether that is really what happened while I stretched, I'm not sure, but the bottom line is it felt good!

Something else I did when I started to get run down was to look at my life and realize how lucky I was. Sometimes I would be in an especially negative attitude, so I would start out with the simplest things that I would often take for granted. For example, no matter what the situation was right then I had a roof over my head, so I would think about how grateful I was for that. I would be grateful for the car I had to drive, and the food I was blessed to eat. Then I would say thank you over and over again for the people in my life who were such blessings.

This became such a powerful process for me that I started waking up early just so I could feel how grateful I was to be living the life I had. Tony Robbins says, "What is wrong is always available. And if there is nothing wrong with you then there is always something wrong with someone you love." But then he also says, "What is right is also always available." This statement is indeed true. If you look for the things that are going to make you feel bad, you will succeed, and vice versa.

The problem is that most of us in our everyday lives have become used to complaining about what is wrong. We tend to focus on the bad and whatever is good we take for granted. It takes practice to every day say thank you for the gift of that day. You have to look at things a little differently to express gratitude for the test that is teaching you to expand your knowledge, use your brain cells, and improve your life in many different ways. There are always different ways of looking at things; sometimes, you need to try a little harder and examine the situation from a different angle.

When you master this skill, you will be able to see the beauty in absolutely everything and every day you will beam with joy!

Another thing that I found very motivating during the hardest times of nursing school was to watch free videos. Many times I really didn't have the extra money to go buy something new for myself. So what I would do was look up some of my mentors' YouTube videos. Anthony Robbins is one of my favorite speakers. What I love about this incredible man is that he motivates you to get things done and to get them done now! What I love about listening to him is that he is constantly sharing his testimony and the testimonies of other successful people. He describes how they were just like us, and the only difference between them is the actions they took. He really puts things in perspective for you.

Another one of my favorite speakers and authors is Deepak Chopra, a medical doctor from India. He is an absolutely wonderful speaker and also has many free YouTube videos. He beautifully describes the miracle of life and how special each of us is. After listening to him, I feel connected to God and have a greater sense of peace.

Marci Shimoff wrote the book *Happy for No Reason*, which made the *New York Times* best seller list. She has a few You Tube videos that are helpful to watch as she describes what it takes to be truly happy. She points out that our goal is not to do more and more to be happy, but to be happy and then out of our love and happiness, take action. You can apply that to your nursing interests by remembering that the goal is to be happy right now, not when you pass nursing school and the NCLEX and have the credentials behind your name.

Joel Osteen is another magnificent speaker. He is able to deliver incredibly positive messages through enlightening speeches and examples that we experience in everyday life. Out of all of the speakers mentioned, he is probably the one with the most free videos available. He also has a TV show on many of the Christian television channels.

Furthermore, if you watch a few of the free YouTube videos and decide you would want to hear more, you can buy the speaker's audio book. Remember that even though time is limited, one hour of inspired studying is worth more than three hours of studying when your heart is simply not into it. I went to Wal-Mart and got a 250 megabyte mp3 player for about $30. It is an iPod for a fraction of the cost. The only drawback is that it doesn't hold as much information. But you can constantly change what is on your device through your computer, or for a little more money, you can get one with more memory.

I went to Audible.com and picked up books from my favorite authors! I selected the book I wanted, the first one of which was, *How to Win Friends and Influence People* by Dale Carnegie. I listened to the book while cleaning the kitchen, vacuuming the house, or washing dishes. Moving around and doing something active while I learned positive ways to improve my life broke up the normal sitting and listening school routine.

It was amazing how much energy I would have after listening to positive words and attitudes for about an hour or two. I had the energy and motivation to get what I needed and wanted done! You see, we all have this voice that is constantly chattering in our heads. This voice is always being influenced by our everyday experiences. If you don't believe that statement, just watch a commercial. If you start brainwashing your mind with positive, motivating information, you won't believe how your life will change for the better.

Furthermore, listening to positive words will give you a sense of purpose. Many of these motivational speakers say the same things in different words. They all believe we were put here for a purpose and that not one second of our day is a mistake. They even point out that, in many instances, our most difficult times end up being the best points of our life, because these are the times that make us ask questions and take actions to make our lives much better.

The next part strategy to keep going strong throughout your nursing education is to simply acknowledge yourself. What do I mean by that? Give yourself some attention! When was the last time you looked into your own eyes and told yourself how much you loved you? If the answer is never, then it is time you start now. I learned from the speakers I mentioned above that many of us don't love ourselves. If we do, we hardly take the time to tell ourselves that.

I started practicing self admiration after I listened to Ms. Shimoff's book. The first time I looked deep into my eyes, it felt weird. I looked away immediately and thought this is so stupid and I was wasting precious studying time. But something inside told me to keep going. So I did it again, this time really looking deep into the pupil of my eye, since I could look at one pupil at a time. With a bewildered and confused look on my face, I said out loud the words that previously had been reserved for others, "I love you, Caroline." The result was astounding, I felt chills over my entire body. I never knew I could have that effect on myself!

Needless to say, I made that practice an integral part of my daily routine. When I brushed my teeth or put on makeup, I would take the time to look at my face, body, and then into my eyes and tell myself how much I loved myself. If you think this is selfish or foolish, remember the Bible says you should love your neighbor as thyself. This already suggests that you love yourself. Give yourself the gift of your own loving attention and admire the truly amazing being that you are.

Another thing that can really keep you going strong throughout the entire nursing school program is the one I found myself skipping over many times. Often I would really feel rundown from all of the constant work. I am speaking about the importance of celebrating your accomplishments! The time after each test is a huge deal; seize the opportunity and celebrate! I'm not sure what celebrating means to you, but to me it meant spending time with family and friends or my boyfriend and dancing, dancing, dancing. I would dance with anyone who would dance with me. If it came down to it, I would even dance with myself in front of my bedroom mirror with my favorite music. Good times!

You must decide what celebrating means to you. Obviously for me, it means bouncing around to my favorite tunes. For you, it could mean watching a movie with a loved one, or going out with your closest friends. It could even mean that you give yourself an hour of meditation, or a bubble bath. Whatever you consider to be fun for you, just make sure you are honest with yourself and don't cheat yourself out of a good time.

Now I have a question for you. How often do you check your email? If you are a good student, then you check your email daily! Imagine every day getting advice from the greatest people who have ever walked this earth. Quotes from people who have been through hard times, who have overcome incredible obstacles. Incredible people leave clues to their success, and the legacy they leave behind in the form of words can inspire and move us!

About three years ago, I started receiving emails from Mark Joyner, a published author who does an internet program called simple-ology. It's an online class that makes you look at your goals, decide what you want and where you are going. He then challenges you to see if you are on the right path. I did his program for a month or two and it was great. That's not why I'm mentioning him, though. The reason I'm bringing this up is because he sends out great daily inspirational quotes. I really like that he sends out a few from the same person, but instead of giving you the name of the individual right away, he asks you to guess who said it.

You find yourself really paying attention to the words, trying to imagine what great person would have said such inspirational things. Then in the third or fourth email, he reveals the person's name. I have only guessed right two times, but I have learned so much by reading these inspirational words every day. You can find this particular program at simpleology.com and sign up for yourself. There are numerous websites that do the same thing. Search in Google "daily inspirational quotes." The best part is that these services are free!

You also may find it important or fulfilling to find ways to serve others. I'm positive since you chose nursing as a career, you are the kind of person who loves to give. Therefore, in order to keep going strong, you may find it powerful to do something for someone else periodically. I found that when I was having negative thoughts about someone -- could be my brother, sister, or parents -- that if I were to do something for them, my negative thoughts would turn into thoughts of love.

Doing something for them doesn't mean you just do something directly and only for that person. It could mean that you clean the kitchen so they will have a nice clean house to live in, or you could vacuum the house and make sure you do their room also. You could cook something they like. You could, of course, buy them a little something or write them a note telling them that you were thinking about them. Sometimes I am sure you feel as if you do not have enough time, or money or even energy. When this is the case and you feel stressed out of your mind, you should still look for an opportunity to help someone else. You will be giving someone a gift, material or nonmaterial, this is true; but in fact, you will be receiving the greatest gift of all.

How to Succeed in Nursing School

Have you noticed that none of the things that I've suggested to keep you motivated in nursing school are directly linked to nursing school? It is really easy to let nursing school dominate your life, but it is also important you take the time to do things for yourself that bring you fulfillment. Remember who you are and why you are pursuing this incredibly challenging degree or license. Then when you feel like you are eating, breathing, and bathing in nursing school, take a deep breath and realize it is time to do something you enjoy. You deserve it!

Caroline Porter Thomas

Chapter 12

The Advantage of Staying Hungry

I like how flexible nursing is. It is a rewarding career and you have interaction with a diverse population.

Madiniah Slaise, RN

Nurse for 1 year Specialty, med-surg and float pool

This may seem oddly placed in a book that is supposed to help you succeed in nursing school. But please read on and keep an open mind. Consider the word "Hungry". Dictionary.com offers a few definitions, one of them being "strongly or eagerly desirous." Isn't it strange we use the same word for when we desire food as when we desire anything else in our lives?

You desire (need) food to stay alive. You can desire to be a nurse for the same reason: to feed, clothe, and provide housing for yourself. The key is to always be hungry, both physically and emotionally, because in a sense they are the same. Have you ever noticed a time when you have tons of energy, then you eat a big meal and cannot even keep your eyes open? Have you ever gone to class after such a massive meal and tried to pay attention? Chances are it was a struggle to keep your eyes open!

Why does this happen? Well, we all know from anatomy and physiology that when we eat food all the blood rushes to the stomach to absorb that food. But if you eat a little side salad and then go to class, it is a totally different experience. You are able to pay attention! The difference is the amount and type of foods you ate. Each satisfied your hunger, but both had profoundly different effects on your body.

What exactly do I mean by staying hungry? I learned this early on when I was in high school and being thin was cool. My friends and my idols were the twigs who walked the runway and posed in magazines. When I felt the slightest bit hungry, I would take immediate action and eat a few bites of something. My hunger was satisfied! Eventually, I realized that I felt better throughout the day when I practiced this. I had great energy levels and was able to do so much more than most people my age.

This included being on the cross country team and working as many as three jobs at one time! After satisfying my hunger with smaller portions, I would go home and be ready to do my homework. Prior to that, I would go home and take two- to three-hour naps! By eating smaller meals more frequently, my grades were better, my social life was better, and my financial life was great! I started getting addicted to my newfound energy. Not only that, I indeed lost weight; it seemed to come off easily and it was fun too.

So the way to be successful at this is to always have healthy snacks around. Some of my favorites are carrots, organic tortilla chips, and a sandwich cut in four pieces. As soon as you feel slightly hungry, quickly satisfy your hunger with a snack, taking small bites, chewing slowly and savoring it. Food is an absolute wonderful thing your body truly needs, so it is important to create positive associations with it. I would always have healthy snacks with me. At the same time, if I found myself craving a particular food, I would do whatever it took to try to get that item immediately, even if it was unhealthy.

For some strange reason, my cravings often consisted of a McDonald's double cheeseburger. Since I told myself that whatever I wanted to eat I would give myself, when that crazy craving came I ate my double cheeseburger. At first, I ate a lot of those double cheeseburgers. But I would eat them in the same way I ate the rest of my food -- always slow and savoring every bite, trying not to finish the whole thing. If I didn't finish, I would bring the leftovers home and sometimes, would finish it later. But more often than not, it found its way into the garbage can.

At first, I ate this junk food all the time, almost once or twice a week. But I found that as I listened to my body, I got these cravings less often. I actually started craving healthier choices, which led me to eating more vegetables as a first line of hunger defense. I think when you tell your body that you cannot have something, you constantly think about that item. After awhile, you give in because it is the only thing on your mind.

When you deny yourself the foods you crave, you may give in and eat large quantities of the item. Do not give up when that happens. Sometimes you may have to train your body repeatedly. The system I just discussed will help you do it. If you keep going, eventually you will make fewer of the unhealthy choices you want to eliminate from your diet. And eventually the amount of times you have meltdowns and eat an entire box of something will become less and less frequent.

Besides eating smaller portions of food very often, another thing that helped improve my overall health and level of energy was eating organic food. The normal foods we are used to eating are often devoid of much of their nutritional properties. If you are interested in learning more about this subject, type "the benefits of an organic diet" on Google and you will find much information. When I started to eat organic foods, I found that I ate smaller quantities, got sick less often, and even my elimination patterns improved.

I think the reason you eat less is because your body is getting the nutrients it needs from a smaller amount of food. If you really listen to your body, you will find that after eating much less food than you normally would, your body will say it has had enough. Although organic food does indeed cost more, will encourage you to eat less. And since you are giving your body the nutrients it needs, you will get sick less. You will save money by not missing work days, or paying for medications and doctor's visits. All together, it may actually save you money in the long run to eat organic foods.

Here is something else I want you to think about. Have you ever eaten three to four apples in a row? This is a weird question, I know. But the next question I want to ask is whether you have ever eaten a whole bag of popcorn, or box of Girl Scout cookies (one of my biggest weaknesses), or drank two Cokes in a row. How are you able to do that? But with apples, or any other fruit for that matter, you do not do that.

The reason for this is because the foods you are able to almost inhale have almost no nutritional properties in them. Your body tries to get the nutrients it needs, so you eat more and more of them. Quickly, the entire bag, box, or drink is gone. Then your body never gets what it needs. Like I said, I am not going to go into too many details about this, but when your body doesn't get what it needs from your foods it will take it from other resources in your body; like your organs. This may keep you alive and going, but it is far from ideal.

I also want to add that many stores are now carrying organic foods at better prices. I have found good selections of organic vegetables, breads and other items at Wal-Mart, Publix, and Food Lion. You may have to search around the store to find them, but it is definitely worth it. If you do live next to a Trader Joe's, Whole foods, or Wild Oats, you are lucky because they have such a great assortment! When you do go shopping, try to stay around the fresh vegetables so you can pack a salad for at least one of your snacks during the day.

Nursing school does indeed induce lots of stress, which is the main reason for emotional eating. You do not need more stress placed on your body by telling yourself you cannot eat something that you want. Then when you finally give in and eat the forbidden item you have desired for so long, you eat four to five times the amount you normally would. If you are like most achievers, which I'm guessing you are or you wouldn't be reading this book; you probably beat yourself up about it. So relax. When the desire comes, satisfy it as soon as you can, and most importantly, enjoy it.

One of the biggest positive disciplines I acquired while in nursing school was to plan my lunches and snacks every day. I always did this the night before. I am sure you have heard the saying, "If you fail to plan, you plan to fail." I know it is corny, but it is so true. Each night before class, I packed my lunch and snacks for the next day. This was such a good habit because first, I packed my food while I was not hungry, so I was able to make wiser choices. I knew that if I woke up and tried to do it in the morning, I would throw anything and everything in there.

Also, I knew that if I did not pack any lunch at all, I would eat fast food all day. This became a ritual for me that I have begun to love. Now that I have graduated and am making a decent amount of money and can afford to eat out every day, I still pack my food for the day. I have even found myself planning my food for the next day when I don't have to go to work. It frees my mind so I can focus on what I am going to accomplish, as opposed to what I am going to feed myself.

Of course, I could not mention a proper diet without stressing the importance of drinking enough water. Researchers say that a lot of times when we feel like we are hungry we are actually thirsty. Our bodies are at least 70% water and if you do not get enough water, your body cannot properly get rid of waste. Instead, it keeps the waste in your body, making you feel tired or sluggish. Also if you drink sodas or juices, you cannot count that as a liquid toward your water amount. Your body really needs 100% pure healthy and natural water, especially without the powdered flavors.

As students, we must sit pretty much all day. Just remember how good it feels when you were sitting in class completely attentive, understanding everything the professor says. Every time you feel the urge to eat something, think to yourself, "Will this make me feel energetic? Or make me feel sleepy?" Then only eat the foods that are going to make you feel good.

Taking care of your body will make your life easier during nursing school and beyond.

Caroline Porter Thomas

Chapter 13

How to Make Nursing School Joyful and Memorable!

We tend to greet each other with the general question, "How are you?" The responses you hear vary, but tend to be negative like, "I'm here," "Just trying to get through the day," and "I'll be happy when this is over." When you watch the news, how often do you see something positive? Sure, news agencies try to share positive uplifting stories occasionally to switch things up a bit, but most news is negative. Pay attention to how rarely you see something positive.

Even commercials are programming you to make you think your life is awful without the product they are trying to sell! We have been programmed to focus on what is wrong in our lives, and this makes it easy to only remember the negative things that happen in nursing school. We tend to look at how hard things are and focus on how difficult our jobs or experiences are. Looking at things in this way is a choice, a matter of perspective. How bad is your life when you look at someone starving in Africa? Suddenly you realize how lucky you are because you have food.

How lucky do you feel that you have read this book? You may feel as if you have a great head start, which you do! How nice was it when a teacher took his/her extra time to help you understand a concept? How great was it when another student went out of his or her way to help you with something? You see, your life could be filled with wonderful memories. The only thing is that you have to work a little harder to notice the good because we are so used to noticing and complaining about the bad.

Try this exercise: Really try it, and don't cheat and look ahead. The first time I did this I was listening to a Tony Robbins audio book. For five seconds, look around and notice everything you can see that is brown......really look! Fast! Fast! Fast! Everything you can see that is brown!

Now close your eyes and say out loud everything you saw that was PINK! Ahhh. I tricked you! You see, if you go looking for the bad things, or the brown in life, you will find it in others and yourself. How do you reprogram yourself to notice everything in your life that is good? Well, honestly, it takes a little practice and determination, but once you start you will feel so good noticing the positive around you that you will get addicted!

One of the first ways I started doing this was to write down five things that happened the day before that made me feel grateful every morning. Physically write them down or type them on the computer. What this will do is make you remember how you felt at that exact moment. Not only that, but whenever you want to feel good, you will have a whole list of things waiting to be read. If possible, I highly recommend you use a computer because then you will never run out of space to write. But, of course, a journal would work as well. You may recognize the name Oprah Winfrey (that was a joke). She recommends doing this on a daily basis. She refers to it as a gratitude journal.

You will notice throughout the day that you begin looking for things to write about in the morning. In those cases, it may be wise to jot down a little note so that you can remember. But this starts reprogramming your mind to look for the good that is out there. When I started doing this, living in an "attitude of gratitude" as they call it, I was completely astonished at how even seemingly insignificant items or events became beautiful. One of the first things I noticed was when I was driving in my car was the sun hitting some leaves on a bush. I was completely speechless as I soaked in all the beauty.

The sun, the bush, and leaves on the bush that I had driven by many times became different that day. I realized all of a sudden that it was because I was noticing the little gifts that God, or whatever you may call your higher power, was offering. This revolutionized my life! I found myself admiring the beauty of my school building that had to be at least 80 years old. I would be so grateful – sometimes to the point of tears -- that it gave me a place to study so I could complete my college education.

Then I would find myself walking through the building and seeing the wonderful things it had to offer. Protection from rain, cold and heat. I felt so grateful for all of these wonderful things. I would get into my car in the morning and feel like I was getting into a Lamborghini or a Rolls Royce, my dream cars. I found myself thanking my car for starting and taking me where I wanted to go. My life felt like a song of joy. And the crazy thing was that nothing had really changed except me, and the way I looked at things. My change in perspective was so powerful that I found I had the energy and right attitude to accomplish any task the instructors put before me. I would even silently thank them for making it challenging because this was a metaphor for my overall life. Imagine how well you would do if every test, assignment, and project was begun with that attitude. The tasks, instead of seeming huge and impossible, were easily broken down and organized into small parts that were easy to do and learn. The attitude you entertain on a daily basis is important to your nursing school experience, but more importantly, it determines the quality of your entire life!

Another way to make nursing school joyful and memorable would be to find a way to help someone at least once a day. Wake up and say to yourself that one of your primary missions of the day is to find someone who needs help! This person could be anyone, and make sure you try to find a way to keep this ritual of yours fun and different. Try and make sure you do something different every day. I'm not saying do not help people you have already helped; just look for others who may need your help also.

Your help may be as simple as cleaning the kitchen for your mom or sitting down to talk with your father about his memories. Most of the time when I see people on the street asking for money I give it, no matter what they are going to do with it. You never know. Maybe that person really is starving and had bad things happen to him. Some of the most successful people I have read about had periods of homelessness and went through times when they could not feed themselves, and they remember the people who helped them. In fact, Conrad Hilton, founder of the Hilton hotels, in his book *Be My Guest*, thanked the bellman who gave him money for food one day.

Of course, I would make it a priority to try and help any of my classmates in any way I could. And I would also make it a priority to try and help my instructors in whatever ways I could also. Many times this involved helping them carry materials to and from class. The important thing to remember in this process, though, is to listen to yourself. I know you want to help others; if not, you would not be in nursing school. However, you must remember to give as much as you can without losing yourself. What I mean by that is always give from a feeling of having plenty for yourself and then give to others so that you can help them feel good too.

I want to share this experience I went through about giving. One day I read the paper and a young gentleman was featured for winning the lottery. I read the story and was, well, jealous. I said to myself, "I would be one of the best candidates to win the lottery." I was thinking about how I would give all of the money in a meaningful way to those who really need it. I would donate to worthy charities, buy my parents the things they dream of, and help my friends through school! I was clearly, a wonderful deserving person to have such a massive amount of wealth to do "good things" with.

Suddenly that voice inside of me also said, "How do I know that? What have you done with what you have already received?" This statement caught me so off guard that at first I defended myself. "What! I haven't received anything! I'm a starving college student!" It was at that moment I realized exactly what I had said. When you focus on what you actually have and you are grateful for it, you will be richer than you could ever imagine. One of the fastest ways to achieve this rich, abundant feeling is to give what you can now. How do you know what you can give now? You would be surprised what you can accomplish with a little planning.

Planning consist of writing down what needs to be done and organizing your time, this is a powerful process. I recommend doing this the night before so that when you open your eyes, you already have instructions and now just need to follow through. By doing this you will be able to consciously think about, even visualize the kind of day you want to have tomorrow. The truth is, you probably already do this. The difference is, you haven't been doing it consciously.

When I started this I was able to accomplish things much faster because instead of waking up and trying to remember everything I had to do, I glanced at the list and took action immediately. In a sense, I was directing how my day would be at the very start. As I wrote down the things I wanted to get done, I visualized myself doing them. For example, when I needed to study for an exam and read a few chapters, I visualized and felt what it feels like to be completely engrossed in studying. Then I would imagine how good I would feel when I was done and completely understood everything. By the time I opened my eyes in the morning I was ready to study, learn or start anything at the top of the list!

This also worked when I had class the next day. I pictured myself in class completely attentive and in total understanding of what my instructor was saying. I would see myself full of energy, able to pay attention and understand the things presented in the classroom with total ease. This process didn't take long. Maybe as long as it took me to write "study med-surg with complete understanding," and I would be done visualizing. Or I would write, "completely understand my instructor," See it, feel it: then I was done.

To ease my mind I would even write the simple things down, so I would not just focus on the big things and forget about the little things. For example, I wrote grab lunch, or water, or even call or text my friend after class. That way I could go to bed with a clear mind, ready to focus on whatever that day brought forth. If you do this even for a little while, I am telling you that you will become addicted! I have done it for three years now, and I am actually at the point where I plan my days off so I can also maximize that time as well!

I have come to realize that being a nursing student and even a nurse, is a title that encompasses only a small portion of my life. So what I do with my "days off" is definitely as important as what I do on my work days. I am committed to using my time in the best way I can and the only way I have found to do that is by planning.

Make sure you plan for the things that are going to help you succeed in class and make your life better. But also make sure you plan to do things that are fun or that allow time with family and friends. Connection with your loved ones is what is really going to give you fulfillment in life. What you do not want to do, though, is spend too much time in one area and suffer for it later. The best way to avoid that is to decide what time of the day is the best for each activity. For studying, you probably need more energy than you do to talk on the phone with a friend.

I discovered I am highly productive in the morning and not so productive in the afternoon. So I would plan to do the hardest things in the morning, which included studying, and then social activities came later in the day. This way I was able to not only maximize my time by knowing what I needed to do the night before but I would also be able to organize the best time to do the activities in a way that my time and energy would be utilized appropriately.

A sample list of your day could look like this. I did not assign times, but if that works for you, do it! Also remember it may seem like a lot at first but as you finish items, check them off, and if any items are remaining you can add them to your list tomorrow.

Caroline Porter Thomas

-Wednesday-

- Wake up feeling rejuvenated and ready to start the day!

- Feel and look my absolute best!

- Grab lunch and water!

- Quickly review the topics to be discussed in class med-surg. 30 minutes GO!!!

- Be ready to learn!

- Study session with Carrie, Cindy, and Rohini!

- Write the outline for my paper in Women's Health!

- Meet with my group to organize our presentation!

- Play with my nieces Katelyn, Abigail, and Sarah!

What you will find is that the more you write down things, plan and schedule, the more you will be able to get done. You'll have extra time because you can also plan and schedule that too. If you really want to make nursing school memorable the key is to organize your time. Realize there are a lot of things that are not fair in this world, but one thing that is equal for all of us is that we each have 24 hours a day, 7 days a week. Plan how you want to use your time, and you will see how nursing school will be a joy.

In conclusion, the best way to think about and appreciate nursing school is to remember that soon enough you will be finished. Successfully, that is! And that these days will eventually come to pass. I know it is hard to imagine because it seems like you are stuck in the classroom with the same people doing the same thing every day. But think back to when you were younger. Didn't you have that feeling before?

I can distinctly remember when my sister got her driver's license. She is seven years older than me and at the time I was far away from ever seeing my driving days. My 9–year-old brain was convinced I would never get a driver's license or ever drive a car.

That day would just never come. But as you and I know, that day came and went and now I drive on a daily basis.

Soon your nursing school experience will pass and the only thing that will be left is the memories you have created. So let's make them good ones. I wish you the best luck in nursing school, and I hope this book helps make your nursing school experience a joyful one!

Power Planning: The One-Week Challenge

Use this guideline to help you focus on your goals and dreams! I started doing power planning three years ago and now I am addicted! I will give you an example of how I use this technique and included room for you to do yours right here in this book!

Here is the outline. I always start with writing how I want to feel in the morning. For example, "Wake up feeling rested and ready to learn!" Directly after that, I write a section where I can record what I am grateful for. I generally put five numbers. Next I write down how I want my character to be that day. I may say, "Today I will look for people who may need some extra help, because I am a loving and giving person." Then I write down my goals or to do's. It looks something like this:

Wake up feeling absolutely wonderful and ready to absorb all information!

Gratitude:

1. I am so grateful that my professors are willing to teach me everything I need to be a successful nurse!

2. I am so grateful that I am constantly reminded of how much I am loved by all the people around me.

3. I am so grateful that I am able to have such positive relationships with my family and friends.

4. I am so grateful for the opportunity of going to nursing school!

5. I am so grateful that I have such a quiet, comfortable area to study so I can accomplish my dreams.

~ Today I want my character to cultivate the art of flexibility and gladly take on any challenge that comes my way ~

Today I am committed to accomplishing:

1. Finishing studying for my OB exam. I see an A!

2. Learn how to safely and effectively insert a foley catheter for clinical.

3. I want to connect with my friend Brittany.

4. Today, I want to find one person who needs a smile... and give it to them!

Now it is your turn! Use this outline for the next seven days and see how your life is going to change immensely!

Day 1

How do you want to feel when you wake up?

_____

What are five things you can be grateful for?

1. _____

2. _____

3. _____

4. _____

5. _____

What kind of person do you want to be today?

_____

What are you committed to accomplishing today?

_____
_____
_____
_____
_____
_____

Day 2

How do you want to feel when you wake up?

_____

What are five things you can be grateful for?

1 _____
2 _____
3 _____
4 _____
5 _____

What kind of person do you want to be today?

_____

What are you committed to accomplishing today?

_____
_____
_____
_____
_____
_____
_____
_____
_____
_____
_____
_____
_____
_____
_____
_____
_____
_____
_____
_____

Day 3

How do you want to feel when you wake up?

_____

What are five things you can be grateful for?

1_____

2_____

3_____

4_____

5_____

What kind of person do you want to be today?

_____

What are you committed to accomplishing today?

_____
_____
_____
_____
_____
_____
_____
_____
_____
_____
_____
_____
_____
_____
_____
_____
_____
_____
_____
_____

Day 4

How do you want to feel when you wake up?

_____

What are five things you can be grateful for?

1 _____

2 _____

3 _____

4 _____

5 _____

What kind of person do you want to be today?

_____

What are you committed to accomplishing today?

_____
_____
_____
_____
_____
_____
_____
_____
_____
_____
_____
_____
_____
_____
_____
_____
_____
_____
_____
_____
_____

Day 5

How do you want to feel when you wake up?

_____

What are five things you can be grateful for?

1_____
2_____
3_____
4_____
5_____

What kind of person do you want to be today?

_____

What are you committed to accomplishing today?

_____
_____
_____
_____
_____
_____
_____
_____
_____
_____
_____
_____
_____
_____
_____
_____
_____
_____
_____
_____
_____

Day 6

How do you want to feel when you wake up?

_____

What are five things you can be grateful for?

1_____

2_____

3_____

4_____

5_____

What kind of person do you want to be today?

_____

What are you committed to accomplishing today?

_____
_____
_____
_____
_____
_____
_____
_____
_____
_____
_____
_____
_____
_____
_____
_____
_____
_____
_____
_____

Day 7

How do you want to feel when you wake up?

_____

What are five things you can be grateful for?

1_____
2_____
3_____
4_____
5_____

What kind of person do you want to be today?

_____

What are you committed to accomplishing today?

_____
_____
_____
_____
_____
_____
_____
_____
_____
_____
_____
_____
_____
_____

Now that you have completed seven days of power planning, it is up to you to decide whether you want to continue doing this. Should you choose to, a small journal would be the best thing for you to use. Also, you might choose to use your computer.

Part 3

After

Chapter 14

Now That You are Finished With Nursing School, Do You Still Need an NCLEX Review?

I love the challenges and opportunity to learn new things. I have worked in so many areas through travel agencies and learned something about most every aspect of nursing. If I had to make a new decision today, I would still choose nursing.

Lori Williams, RN

Specialty: Many different ones/ ER – present

Yes... you still need a NCLEX review.

Shereta Jones' inspiring story of persistence

"You never quite prepare yourself for taking NCLEX. You think you are preparing the entire time you're in school, but once you graduate and begin to study you see that everything does not work out as planned. I graduated May 10, 2008. When you're in school you cannot wait for this day, but it is only the beginning of the journey. I sat there and listened to the long speeches thinking it was finally over; I graduated from college with a Bachelors of Science in Nursing. Then it dawned on me -- I am still not finished.

"I still had to take NCLEX. I mapped out a plan. I will attend NCLEX reviews and study, and then take NCLEX the second week in June. I figured I would be well prepared by then, but I was sadly mistaken. The second week of June came, and I was still studying and attending another NCLEX review. I felt I wasn't prepared yet, so I kept studying, attending NCLEX reviews and doing that famous task that nursing instructors tell you to do: questions. I felt like there was so much I didn't know or understand after all those years of school and studying. I thought to myself, 'Will I ever be ready to take this test?' July approached and I made up in my mind to take this test. I didn't tell a soul I was going to do it, not even my two best friends I met while attending nursing school. But I broke down and told my Mom I was going to take the test. She drove me to the test, and I was so nervous.

"I have never been a good test taker but I still felt I was prepared enough. I went in nervous and anxious and when I sat down to take the test, my fingers began to tremble. I prayed for strength and knowledge as I began to answer questions. Unfortunately, it was like another language; the questions were so much more complex in comparison to the questions I practiced during my studying. I pressed on through the test. The screen went blank right after I answered the 75th question and all I could think was 'Thank you, God, this is over.'

"I left the testing site still nervous and anxious, but also happy it was over and I could get my life back that I had been missing the last couple of years. I took the test on a Wednesday so that meant my results would be ready on Friday. Thursday came and I couldn't contain my self. I called the two best friends anyone could ever ask for to tell them I had taken the test.

"They were happy and supportive. They praised me with positive comments, saying I did well and that I was already a nurse. Talking to them made me feel so much better about myself, and it gave me confidence that I had passed. Friday came and I logged on to the Internet to check my status. As I began to put in my pass codes and credit card information, my fingers were shaking and I could feel my heart beating in my ears. I was so nervous. Then I scrolled down and saw fail. I was in shock. I felt like someone had just stolen my world. I cried and cried. I didn't have the heart right then to call and talk to my friends so I sent them a text message. The message read: 'Please don't be discouraged or disappointed. I did not pass.'

"It was a horrible time for me, but I got the strength to keep pushing myself. I picked back up on my studying and attended a few more sessions of NCLEX reviews. I did question after question and told no one of my first attempt at NCLEX but my friends and my Mom. They kept me encouraged and motivated. I chose other dates to take my test and kept seeing 'fail' pass before my eyes. And I would change the date frequently. However, I kept studying and practicing NCLEX questions. I had done over 4,000 questions and figured I was ready to take the test again. I did not keep it to myself that I was going to take the test. I told everyone who would listen, and I asked for their prayers. This time my two best friends and I were going to take the test around the same time. I made the attempt first. At the end of September, I went on a Wednesday to the same location as in July. I walked in nervous and anxious, and as I began to take the test, I thought to myself, 'Where do they get these questions? I have never seen this stuff before in my life.'

"I approached 75 questions and the computer did not shut off. I thought, 'OK, I am doing a little better but please don't give me too many more questions.' I made it to 100 questions then 150 then 200. When I reached 200, my mind was shot; I couldn't go on even with the breaks. I received the whole 275 questions and it took me from 8 a.m. to 1 p.m.. I felt betrayed, as if I had done all those questions for nothing because I still didn't feel like I knew anything on that entire test. One of my friends from nursing school had driven me to the testing site this time, so when I got in the car, I felt so overwhelmed all I wanted to do was cry. I couldn't even talk without being forced into tears. But she wouldn't allow it. I had a horrible feeling about the test this time. I felt like I had bombed that test, but once again my friends were there with support and positive remarks, which boosted my confidence.

"I checked my results Friday, but they weren't ready. I called back on Saturday, waiting through the voice recording shaking and trembling. Then I heard, 'You did not pass your NCLEX examination.'

"Words cannot describe the way I felt. I had to call back again to see if I heard correctly. I was back to square one. This time, it wasn't easy to jump back on the study bandwagon. I was devastated. In fact, I think I was more devastated this time around than the first. My two best friends went on to take the test and passed on the first try. I was thrilled they passed because I knew there would be hope for me, after all. I started reviewing Judith Miller tutorials and completed the entire set. I did not do many questions on this third round of studying. I listened to the tutorials and took notes. In all, I don't think I completed a 1,000 questions.

"I had so much anxiety and self doubt about this third attempt. But, if the inevitable should happen again, I made up my mind that I would find strength to study and retake it again. I had come too far to turn around and, even though the odds and statistics were against me, I pushed on. I finally got up enough courage to schedule a date and stick with it. I set my appointment for January 8, 2009, and made sure it was not on a Wednesday. I had had enough of Wednesday testing. I also scheduled this test outside my home state of North Carolina. I scheduled it in the state of South Carolina, which had become my second home in my time of studying. I woke up late, but was still on time for my 8 a.m. test.

"I went in to take the test and, for the first time, felt a sense of comfort. I didn't know all of the questions, but I felt I knew some of them. My computer got to 75 and it did not shut off. Anxiety crept back in, but I said a prayer and kept pushing. The last time I looked at the question number I was on 80 something. My computer shut down not long after that; I know it didn't make it to 100. I panicked for a second. I wanted more time.

"When I left, I didn't feel the normal anxiety and nervousness. I felt a sense of comfort. Two days later, which was Saturday, January 10, 2009, I went on the testing website to check my results. Once again, I was nervous while checking them and when I saw 'pass' all I could do was cry and cry and tell everyone. I couldn't call or text fast enough to tell them my good news. I was overjoyed. I think I cried all day Saturday, and I still get a little choked up when I talk about it. My hard work paid off. I accomplished such a big goal in my life. I never gave up because that was not an option; I just prayed and kept moving.

"So my message to new grads, nursing students, and those thinking about becoming a nurse is; **NEVER GIVE UP**. The road is rough and it is not easy at all, but keep pushing and praying and you can accomplish and be so much in life. I passed the NCLEX and you can too!"

Shereta Jones, BSN, RN

Fayetteville State University

My Story

"When it was time for me to graduate nursing school, I told my mother I didn't want to celebrate with a party. I explained that my degree was worth nothing unless I passed the licensing board examination. My mom got her way, and we had a nice party anyway. I have to admit it was nice to celebrate making it this far, and I enjoyed it thoroughly. Directly following the party, I switched back into serious mode. I said every day to myself, 'Wow, you passed in 75 questions. You are so intelligent!' In my head over and over while I was studying, I said this to myself.

"I was blessed to attend a school that provided us with NCLEX reviews. I attended every single one, every single day. I noticed many of my classmates taking vacations or simply taking time off from studying. I often wondered why, as our four years meant nothing without passing this final licensing exam. After the review every day, I went home and studied what we had gone over that day. In my head still, 'Wow, you passed in 75 questions. You are so intelligent!'

"I signed up to take my exam the first date I could, which happened to be a month after graduation. I was surprised to see that I could sign up for a two o'clock test time. As I like to sleep in, this was the time I chose. I also found a job at Central Carolina Hospital that allowed me to follow an RN before I passed the board examination, and get paid while doing so. On the days I didn't have a NCLEX review or follow my RN, I allowed myself only one luxury. This was to sleep in until 10 am. Once awake, I made myself repeat question after question. I still repeated in my head, 'Wow, you passed in 75 questions. You are so intelligent!'

"Two weeks before my exam, I was introduced to Pearson VUE. This company had NCLEX review questions on the computer. Every morning I answered question after question. In the evenings I would go over questions I didn't understand with my mother, the nurse. She would help me understand the rationale or help me look up the answer. In those two weeks, I completed every single question on that website. Sometimes in the mirror I would say to myself, 'Wow, you passed in 75 questions. You are so intelligent!'

"Many of my NCLEX review instructors suggested taking a few days off before your exam so you would not be too stressed out. Some of my classmates did this and it worked perfectly for them. I knew myself and realized I wasn't comfortable with that. During my entire time in nursing school I studied until my instructor told me to close my book. For the last most important exam, I was not about to change my strategy. Again and again, 'Wow, you passed in 75 questions. You are so intelligent!'

"Two days before the exam I drove to the location of the exam. I wanted to make sure I knew exactly where to go on 'the day.' I went home and again repeated question after question. I still allowed myself only one luxury of sleeping in until about 10 a.m. because I was able to get a 2 p.m. test time. I knew I could also do this on test day. While driving back home, I kept looking in the mirror saying to myself, 'Wow, the test shut off in 75 questions. You know what that means!'

"Test day. I woke up at 10 a.m. just like I planned. I went through my morning routine of telling myself, 'Wow, you passed in 75 questions, you are so intelligent!' I ate breakfast while still doing more questions. Time flew and before I knew it I was driving to my test location.

"Fear suddenly came over me. I thought, "Oh, I need something to make me feel better or give me some energy." Right away I pulled into the nearest gas station, tires screeching and all. I went straight for a Mountain Dew. It had been so long since I drank one, possibly five years, but when I consumed them before I was always buzzing off of a sugar and caffeine high for hours. I drank it immediately and continued onto my destination. By this time, I was practically screaming, 'Wow, you passed your NCLEX exam in 75 questions!'

"I arrived at the location about an hour early. I began looking over notes, my nerves, however, would not let me comprehend anything I was reading. I looked over these notes for 30 minutes then finally went inside the building to take the test. The test room was much smaller than I was expecting, and there was almost no one in sight. I expected to be in a crowded room with many more nursing students about to take their exams. However, it was nothing like that.

"I was early, but it didn't matter. I went right up to the counter, handed the person my test information and my driver's license, then posed for my photo. They gave me a locker for my sweater and said 'Okay, you can go ahead.' As I went up to the exam room, I was closely examined by the proctor who asked me what the bump in my pocket was. 'Ummm, I'm not sure.' I reached into my pocket to find my ChapStick. I was told to put that in my locker as well.

"When I came back, I was told the rules of the room. I was given a small dry-erase board if I needed to write anything down. I was told I could have as many bathroom breaks as necessary; I simply needed to raise my hand and the proctor would lead me out. I then was led to my cubby, which had my computer on it. I entered all of the information it asked, and then answered three example questions. I was told at one of my reviews these example questions would determine the level of difficulty your questions would begin at.

How to Succeed in Nursing School

"Question one. The question came up but I couldn't see it! My heart was beating out of my chest and I felt like I was going to pass out! 'Maybe the Mountain Dew wasn't such a good idea. Oh my gosh, what if I fail my exam!' Panic-stricken, I sat there, unable to read the first question and drowning in fear. 'Breathe, Caroline,' I said calmly to myself. 'Just breathe, slowly, easily. If you don't pass, you can take it again. Everything will work out.'

"It felt like five minutes that I was breathing and talking calmly to myself. The clock however said 30 seconds. I finally blinked one last time and was able to read the question. Question after question came. They were so difficult, just like I imagined. I did every question just like I always practiced, reading, rereading, then reading the answers, then again rereading the question. Then finally, selecting what I thought was the most appropriate choice.

"I went though each question like this. The majority of my questions were med-surg based. I was pretty nervous about this, because this had been my hardest course while I was in school. I kept getting "select all that apply" questions, too, which I always thought were so difficult. I had to do breathing exercises several times during the exam. As the numbers began to rise, I had to make myself breathe slowly even more.

"73, 74, 75. I looked at the number 75 for about 30 seconds before I could even read the question. I read, reread, then looked at the answers, then again reread the question. At one of my reviews I was told that if you remember the last question you had and you knew you got it right, you probably passed. I selected my answer and tried desperately to remember this question. Every time I was about to press the submit key I completely forgot the question.

"I did this several times before I finally said to myself, 'Caroline, if you have to do more questions, it's OK.' I talked myself into truly believing that and breathed some more as I pressed the submit key. The computer screen went blank. 'Oh no! I didn't remember the last question! Did I pass? Did I fail?' The whole time I imagined myself taking this exam I saw myself feeling so confident afterwards. I felt nothing of the sort.

"Driving home I could hardly talk. My nursing school friends called me and assured me that I passed. I didn't feel as good as I wanted though. Over the next few days, while waiting for my results,

I just didn't feel that great. When the third day came and I was able to go online to see my results I was so nervous to do so.

"I sat in the living room with my Mom and Dad. I went to the website, put in my information and waited for what seemed like an eternity. I was concentrating so hard on the screen I didn't even notice my parents disappeared. Finally, it came up and said my result in tiny little 12 point font! 'pass.' 'I passed!' I exclaimed! My parents came into the kitchen carrying a cake that said, "Caroline Porter BSN-RN" and a bottle of champagne!

"As proud as I was that I passed my exam in 75 questions, not one person besides my classmates ever asked me that question. My boss didn't care what my grades in school were and when I got my license, they were just happy I could work as an RN. Bottom-line, no matter how many questions or times you take the exam, pass is pass. In the end you're a licensed or registered nurse. That is all they care about. I have come to find out myself that is really all that matters as well."

Chapter 15

The Unlimited Growth Possibilities

Are you happy with your decision to become a nurse?

Yes, I feel called to nursing. My mom has a questionnaire from elementary school where I wrote I wanted to be a nurse. I never really had to choose a career. I always knew I loved science and wanted to take care of people. It made my college choices very easy! I think to pick nursing as a career for the money or the hours would be difficult because it's a very hard job. You have to be committed to working hard and not getting discouraged. Some experiences are very challenging but the relationships you form with patients and their families make it all worthwhile.

If you had to make a new decision today would you chose nursing?

Yes, I would. I think that every day is a challenge and that being in the float pool gives you a great opportunity to start each day fresh, to be prepared to work hard, and to learn as much as you can. The 'on-the-job training' with nursing never ends! There are patients I had two years ago that I can still remember their names and specific conversations we had. As much as I hope to touch my patients' lives and to teach them, they teach me so much more. Even a difficult patient is like any other person. If you look hard enough you can find the good in them and in the situation. I love laughing with my patients and their families.

A nurse is the patient's link to having their needs met, getting answers to their questions, understanding their diagnosis, and learning how to care for themselves at home. The bond of trust between a patient and their nurse is something to truly be appreciated.

Alyson Bond – RN for 2 years

Specialty, Intermediate ICU/float pool

The person who chooses nursing as a career places him or herself in a position with seemingly unlimited potential for growth. This is so enticing to the individual who wants to accomplish a lot in his or her life! In this chapter I will give you an example of different positions in the hospital setting. After that we will explore advance degrees, and more. Once you have graduated, the first position in a hospital that most new nurses work is as a floor nurse in their chosen specialty. In the past, units like the ICU or labor and delivery would not hire new grads until they had at least a year in med-surg. However, this has changed in many hospitals with new graduates beginning in the ED or ICU.

When you have proven yourself competent in your specialty, the next step would be to train other nurses as their preceptor. This does not pay much more, but one advantage of teaching others is that you also will learn many new things and become much more competent yourself. Also realize that it is flattering to be able to train others. This means your employer recognizes your competence. Keep in mind that the administration will be watching the fruit of your labor closely. If you train your preceptee well, proving your success in this position, increased responsibilities will be offered to you, and you will surely be invited to the interview for the next higher level position. For instance, you may be considered for a "charge nurse" position. Some places refer to this nurse as resource nurse or clinical leader. Whatever the title is, generally this person is responsible for monitoring the nursing care given by all the nurses and aides on the unit. Also, the charge nurse must stay abreast of each patient's condition under his/her charge. They also must be sure there is adequate staff to care for the patients. She or he must be available to help the nurses with procedures they may need assistance with, educating the staff as necessary.

Being a charge nurse is quite different then being a floor nurse. You must look at things such as the acuity of the patient. Acuity means how much nursing care a patient requires. A patient who can walk, talk and care for their basic needs, would be a low acuity patient. Compare that to a patient who cannot even lift her arm, or feed herself. These high acuity patients require close monitoring and more frequent checks. In many cases, one high acuity patient could be equivalent to having two to four low acuity patients when you look at the nursing care needs.

The charge nurse is also responsible for assessing the number of patients each nurse has. He or she must take into consideration the nurses' ability to care for the patients. This position requires monitoring of all procedures, policies, and physician orders. As a charge nurse, you would be in close communication with the emergency department and other areas of the hospital in regards to admissions. When a room is available, you will inform the floor nurse that they will be getting a new patient and assist that nurse in any way needed.

Once you have been a charge nurse for awhile, you may want to work as the nurse manager or hospital director. The nurse manager is responsible for the hiring and firing of staff and creating the schedule, amongst other administrative duties that vary from hospital to hospital. The nursing director is the one who oversees all the nursing operations of the hospital. His or her other main responsibility is making sure there is enough staff coming in when the census is high, and controlling staffing when the census is low. The hospital director generally does not partake in direct patient care.

The people who address patient's insurance questions and make sure the nurses are appropriately documenting are called case managers. This title involves much paperwork and time talking on the phone to various agencies such as nursing homes. The case manager speaks with the patient and/or family if there is a concern related to cost or insurance. They also help make sure the patients who are well enough to go home do so, and they make preparations for any care or equipment needed in the home setting. At first, this position may not sound appealing, but after years on your feet and for someone who may no longer be interested in direct patient care, it can become more attractive.

There are many more positions available to motivated nurses. The positions that I have mentioned, thus far, are in the hospital setting. Of course, other options are available, but they are not as well known and vary from place to place. Know that other opportunities are out there for the LPN or RN. Another way to continue on the path upward is to further your education. For the LPN or associate degree RN you could complete requirements to obtain a bachelors' degree in nursing. This will help you get into management more quickly (if it is not already a requirement), and in most hospitals you will also get paid more.

Advance degree nursing opens many exciting opportunities. The initial requirement is a bachelor's degree. There are four main types of nursing advanced degrees. I will give you a very brief description of each. The first is called the nurse practitioner's license. Nurse practitioners are given more freedom than the general nurse. For example, nurse practitioners have the ability to prescribe drugs. They can practice independently or alongside physicians. They usually see common uncomplicated patients in their chosen population. The main populations to choose from as a nurse practitioner are the general adult population, the geriatric population, and the pediatric population.

A geriatric nurse practitioner treats the elderly population, usually ages 65 and older. With the baby boomers advancing in age there will be a great need for geriatric nurse practitioners in the next 10 to 20 years. The pediatric nurse practitioner treats the common uncomplicated problems in children ages 18 and younger. As a nurse practitioner, you could also treat entire families. The family nurse practitioner could see their patients on a regular basis and help them manage their illnesses and educate them about their health for optimal wellness. There are still other nurse practitioner specialties, but these are the main ones.

This next master's degree is called the nurse anesthetist. A nurse anesthetist is the person who manages anesthesia for surgical patients or other invasive procedures. This degree is much sought after as the average starting salary is six figures. If you go to a rural hospital you could be starting in the 120's. This certification, however, does not come easily. Nurse anesthetist school is an intense 2+ years. Most of the programs don't even allow you to work while you attend their program. Also, acceptance into these programs is very competitive, so having a very high GPA in your undergraduate classes and at least one year of experience in an ICU is imperative.

If you are the type of nurse who loves maternal labor and delivery, you may want to consider obtaining the nurse midwife license. If you have ever seen a delivery, you know how special it is to be with parents the first time they see their child. It truly is a magic moment. Imagine sharing that magic moment with mothers all the time while you assist in the delivery of their newborns. Nurse midwives assist in the uncomplicated deliveries. They can also see the expecting mothers for their checkup visits.

The final nursing advance degree I will discuss is the nurse educator. This master's degree gives you the option of teaching nursing courses at the college level. Your MSN alone may be enough to get your foot in the door at many community colleges and possibly at a university. Most colleges require a Doctorate although many colleges will employ you under the contingency that you will be working toward it. Many nurse educators that I know worked as a nurse for years and then chose to specialize in nursing education. It is not unheard of to go straight from your bachelor's, work for a year, and then get your advance degree to educate others.

If you are not ready to go back to school for your bachelor's or master's degree right away, there are many certificate options. Once you have a few years working in your selected area, you can look at the options available to you. You can explore the directory online at www.testprepreview.com/nursing_certifications.htm. Here they offer online preparation information. They do list the master's degree programs that I mentioned above, but the majority of the certifications can be obtained without getting your master's.

This site tells you what the requirements are for the certifications. Most of the requirements start out with the time you need to be working in the specialty area and how many CEUs or continuing education units (hours) you need. Most hospitals provide plenty of CEU hours for free, and some that are optional to pay for. Many of these certifications may be obtained in a matter of days once you have met the requirements, although some take longer. Examples are: Certified Dialysis Nurse (CDN), Certified Neuroscience RN (CNRN), Oncology Certified Nurse (OCN), Sexual Assault Nurse Examiner (SANE), Certified Ostomy Care Nurse (COCN), Certified Infection Control Nurse (CIC), Certified Emergency Nurse (CEN), and many more. These certifications look great on your resume and make you highly marketable.

The final choice that I am going to present in a mini summary for you is "travel nursing." Travel nursing is when you work for a company that will assist you in obtaining a temporary job in a different location; one that may be appealing to you. You can select the hospital, or the area you want to work and they will provide you with a place to live. Travel nursing is much more profitable than just doing regular staff nursing. You normally work in 13-week assignments, where you work three standard 12-hour shifts. You get to travel, see the country or even the world, get paid a premium wage, and you do not have to pay rent! Normally, at least one to two years of experience in a chosen specialty is required. Assignments can pay anywhere from $25 to $60 an hour depending on your experience and travel location.

As you can once again see, nursing has boundless opportunities. I want you to make a promise to me. If you find yourself unhappy at your job, change it. There are so many different things you can do with your license that you are selling yourself short by spending one minute in a place where you are not happy. Some of us can work in the same place for years and years. Many people need constant change. There is nothing wrong with either one. Do what feels right, but most importantly, have fun as a nurse!